More Advance Praise for

Pain

"It was a pleasure to read the advance copy of *Pain* in the "What do I do now" series. Drs. Washington, Brown, and Fanciullo do an admirable job of condensing the field of pain medicine into important clinical vignettes which bring the reader effortlessly through complex, interesting cases using 'best practices' in pain medicine. The highly readable volume is rationally divided into three sections: chronic pain conditions, chronic pain related disorders, and treatment overview. In my opinion, the chapters on the difficult pain patient and medical marijuana are among the best I have seen anywhere. This book will serve the busy primary care practitioner and the pain specialist alike with helpful clinical pearls throughout."

—*Allen W. Burton, MD, Houston Pain Associates, Houston, TX*

"This eighth volume of the new series entitled "What Do I Do Now?" by Drs. Tabitha A. Washington, Khalilah M. Brown, and Gilbert J. Fanciullo covers a wide variety of challenging clinical pain syndromes as well as the latest therapies. The authors elegantly present each case with a comprehensive yet clinically relevant review of the literature in order to provide the reader with a rapid and clear understanding of chronic pain conditions as well as the most appropriate therapeutic options. The expertise of the authors is put in the practicing clinician's hands though an attractive format of tables, figures, references and bullet points. This also makes it attractive for exam preparation."

—*Thomas T. Simopoulos, MD, MA, Director of the Interventional Pain Service, Arnold Pain Management Center, Beth Israel Deaconess Medical Center, Boston, MA*

"Chronic pain is complex and difficult to treat, and often leaves clinicians perplexed about what to do when usual analgesics fail. 'What do I do now?' *Pain* directs readers through a variety of scenarios, clinical cases that represent common chronic pain diagnoses (section 1), linked disorders (section 2), and different treatment types (section 3). The format is easy to follow, and key points at the end of each chapter focus the lessons learned through each case. Washington, Brown and Fanciullo are recognized authorities and have produced a book that will appeal to a wide range of practitioners, regardless of specialty."

—*Jane C. Ballantyne, MD, FRCA, Professor of Anesthesiology and Pain Medicine, Center for Pain Relief, University of Washington, Seattle, WA*

What Do I Do Now?

SERIES CO-EDITORS-IN-CHIEF

Lawrence C. Newman, MD
Director of the Headache Institute
Department of Neurology
St. Luke's-Roosevelt Hospital Center
New York, NY

Morris Levin, MD
Co-director of the Dartmouth Headache Center
Director of the Dartmouth Neurology Residency Training Program.
Section of Neurology
Dartmouth Hitchcock Medical Center
Lebanon, NH

PREVIOUS VOLUMES IN THE SERIES

Headache and Facial Pain
Peripheral Nerve and Muscle Disease
Pediatric Neurology
Stroke
Epilepsy
Neurocritical Care
Neuro-Ophthalmology
Neuroimmunology

Pain

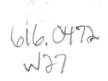

Tabitha A. Washington, MD, MS
Associate Pain Fellowship Program Director, Section of Pain Medicine
Department of Anesthesiology
Dartmouth Hitchcock Medical Center
Dartmouth Medical School
Lebanon, NH

Khalilah Brown, MD, MPH
Department of Anesthesiology
Dartmouth Hitchcock Medical Center
Lebanon, NH

Gilbert Fanciullo, MD, MS
Director, Section of Pain Medicine
Department of Anesthesiology
Dartmouth Hitchcock Medical Center
Dartmouth Medical School
Lebanon, NH

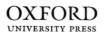
OXFORD
UNIVERSITY PRESS

OXFORD
UNIVERSITY PRESS

Oxford University Press, Inc., publishes works that further Oxford University's objective of excellence in research, scholarship, and education.

Oxford   New York
Auckland   Cape Town   Dar es Salaam   Hong Kong   Karachi   Kuala Lumpur   Madrid
Melbourne   Mexico City   Nairobi   New Delhi   Shanghai   Taipei   Toronto

With offices in
Argentina   Austria   Brazil   Chile   Czech Republic   France   Greece   Guatemala   Hungary   Italy
Japan   Poland   Portugal   Singapore   South Korea   Switzerland   Thailand   Turkey   Ukraine   Vietnam

Published by Oxford University Press, Inc.
198 Madison Avenue, New York, New York 10016
www.oup.com

First issued as an Oxford University Press paperback, 2012

Library of Congress Cataloging-in-Publication Data

Washington, Tabitha A.
Pain/Tabitha A. Washington, Khalilah Brown, Gilbert Fanciullo.
     p. ; cm.—(What do I do now?)
Includes bibliographical references and index.
ISBN 978-0-19-982760-2 (pbk. : alk. paper)
1. Pain—Diagnosis—Case studies.   2. Pain—Treatment—Case studies. I. Brown, Khalilah. II. Fanciullo, Gilbert. III. Title. IV. Series: What do I do now?
[DNLM: 1. Pain—diagnosis—Case Reports.   2. Pain—therapy—Case Reports.   3. Diagnosis, Differential—Case Reports. WL 704]
RB127.W37 2012
616'.0472   dc23
2011026018

The science of medicine is a rapidly changing field. As new research and clinical experience broaden our knowledge, changes in treatment and drug therapy occur. The author and publisher of this work have checked with sources believed to be reliable in their efforts to provide information that is accurate and complete, and in accordance with the standards accepted at the time of publication. However, in light of the possibility of human error or changes in the practice of medicine, neither the author, nor the publisher, nor any other party who has been involved in the preparation or publication of this work warrants that the information contained herein is in every respect accurate or complete. Readers are encouraged to confirm the information contained herein with other reliable sources, and are strongly advised to check the product information sheet provided by the pharmaceutical company for each drug they plan to administer.

Printed in the United States of America
on acid-free paper

#732776442

To my Michael, thank you for all your love and support. To our children, Gwendolyn and Ethan, who are my inspiration in everything I do and every choice I make. To my parents, James and Alice, who have always supported me in every endeavor and made me who I am today. To my family, who have always been there for me, and have never doubted my dreams. In loving memory of my father, James Ethan Washington.

—*TW*

To Delores and Jesse, who inspire and encourage my every step and whom without fail and with more love than any one person deserves. To Sallie, my conscience; Krystal, my spirit; and Patrick, my heart—I stand on your shoulders. Thank you.

—*KB*

To Peggy. Thank you, Darling, for your sacrifices, support, and love.

—*GF*

Preface

Chronic Pain is a debilating disorder which is often difficult to treat. Diagnosis can be complex, patients' can be time consuming for practioners and treatment may seem futile. It is the practioner whom often first encounters these patients and when treatment is unsuccessful will often ask, "What do I do now?" Literature review and textbooks can be helpful, however time consuming and expansive for the practioner to utilize in their busy practices which are limited by time and financial constraints. A quick resource could help facilitate treatment of chronic pain patients.

This book was developed as a tool to allow the reader to recognize and appropriately treat a variety of pain disorders using a case study format. The cases used are derived from both inpatient and outpatient consultation requests from providers in medical practice. We have divided the book into 3 sections to address common topics that one may encounter in the pain patient; (1) Chronic pain conditions (2) Chronic pain and related disorders and (3) Treatment overview. Each chapter is written utilizing the most up to date information. Tables are included to allow for representation of written material. Key points are included at the end of each chapter to summarize.

This book is designed as a resource for all practioners who treat pain, as it provides a succinct and logical approach to diagnosis and management of painful conditions encountered frequently in medical practice.

Tabitha Washington
Hanover, NH

Contents

SECTION I CHRONIC PAIN CONDITIONS

1 **Complex Regional Pain Syndrome** 1
Commonly over diagnosed, CRPS has little especial association with the
Autonomic Nervous System, does not involve Dystrophy, and has no known
Reflex associated with it. Type 1 is the classical Reflex Sympathetic Dystrophy
differing from Type 2- Causalgia, only in that Type 2 involves injury to a major
nerve.

2 **Peripheral Neuropathy** 10
The debilitating pain of peripheral neuropathy can be difficult to treat and relies
on pain management and treatment of the underlying pathology. This chapter
reviews the causes, sign and symptoms, diagnostic criteria and treatment options
available for these patients.

3 **Postherpetic Neuralgia** 16
Post-herpetic neuralgia is a devastating and painful consequence of shingles
(herpes zoster) and is most common in the elderly and the immunocompromised.
Medications are the mainstay of treatment, however caution should be used in
the elderly secondary to side effects.

4 **Central Post-Stroke Pain** 22
Often thought only in association with thalamic pain syndrome following infarct
to the thalamus, pain following stroke may occur with any setting of stroke
affecting nociceptive fibers at any level. Neuropathic or central pain can occur in
up to 8% of patients after a stroke. Medical treatment usually begins with a trial
of Lamotrigine and a second-line drug may be added. For severe, refractory cases,
repetitive transcranial magnetic stimulation (rTMS) may be offered.

5 **Multiple Sclerosis Related Pain** 29
Multiple sclerosis (MS) is usually associated with a loss of sensation; however,
since the late 1800s, physicians have recognized that pain is often associated
with multiple sclerosis and can at times be the heralding symptom. Pain can
occur in 29-86% of MS patients an can include neuropathic pain, dysesthetic
pain and trigeminal neuralgia, as well as somatic pain mostly originating from
back pain and painful spasms. Medication, physical therapy, behavioral therapy,
occupational therapy, interventional procedures, baclofen pump placements, and
surgical interventions have been employed.

6   **Radiculopathy**   35
Probably the most common cause of neuropathic pain, lumbar and cervical
radiculopathy are frequently encountered clinical entities while thoracic is
more rare. These syndromes may involve an anatomical abnormality and can be
gratifying to both diagnose and treat, but a nonanatomical abnormality syndrome
is equally as common and presents more of a diagnostic and therapeutic dilemma
or even conundrum.

7   **Brachial Plexus Injury**   39
Brachial plexus injuries are most commonly due to trauma, of which, motor cycle
accidents are the most common. Men are most frequently affected. Other causes
can include; penetrating or sports related injuries, falls, work related accidents,
radiation therapy and iatrogenic causes (ie, first rib resection, shoulder surgery,
interventional radiology). The most common mechanism of injury is a traction
injury due to forceful separation of the neck from the shoulder. Persistent brachial
plexus pain is often treated in a fashion similar to neuropathic pain.

8   **Superficial Radial Nerve Injury**   46
This small sensory nerve can be a cause of excruciating pain when injured
iatrogenically. Diagnosis can be confusing and treatment a challenge.

9   **Post-Thoracotomy Pain (Acute and Chronic Pain)**   49
Persistent post-thoracotomy pain syndrome (PTPS) is one of the most prevalent
sources of chronic post-operative pain. Up to 20-70% of patients may complain
of symptoms consistent with post-thoracotomy pain. Targeting the points
before, during, and after surgery that could decrease the risk of PTPS has been
understudied and there is no clear evidence for any specific recommendations.
That being said, recommendations and standard of care include a multimodal
analgesic approach during surgery and perioperatively with nonopioid and
local anesthesia. Treatment of chronic PTPS can include medical therapy,
interventional therapy and in those with refractory disease, spinal cord
stimulation.

10   **Dental Pain**   53
Branches of the Trigeminal Nerve are not infrequently injured during routine dental
procedures and can produce symptoms similar to Tic Douloureux. Proper anatomical
localization and an understanding of the mechanism of injury can be important
considerations in selecting treatment approaches or determining prognosis.

11   **Trigeminal Neuralgia and Atypical Facial Pain**   57
Trigeminal neuralgia is a debilitating disease that affects a subset of patients. This
chapter focuses on the epidemiology, diagnostic criteria and management of
patients. Special considerations to the elderly population who are at higher risk of
developing side effects from treatment.

12 **Phantom Pain** 62

Phantom pain is described as pain or dysesthesia that is caused by interruption or discontinuation of sensory nerve impulses by destroying or injuring the sensory nerve fibers after amputation or deafferentation. The usual cause of pain is due to trauma or surgical manipulation. The incidence of phantom limb pain varies across studies and is on the order of 2-80%; however, the average appears to be between 40-70%. Medical therapy should be tried initially and should not be considered a failure until narcotic therapy has been trialed. Surgical therapy including spinal cord stimulator placement and DREZ lesions should be reserved for refractory cases.

13 **Spinal Cord Injury and Pain** 65

Injury to the spinal cord can occur via trauma, infection, ischemia, toxicity, tumor, radiation, disease or other causes. The pattern of pain may still be changing years or even decades after injury. The level of pain and disability may be very high and effective treatment options may be illusory.

14 **Ramsey Hunt Syndrome (Geniculate Neuralgia)** 69

Ramsay- Hunt Syndrome is a rare entity that was first described in the early 1907 by James Ramsay Hunt. There are three Ramsay-Hunt Syndromes that vary dramatically from one another with the only similarity being that they were described by the same person. In this article, we will discuss Ramsay Hunt Syndrome Type II, commonly known as herpes zoster oticus and is accompanied by a peripheral facial palsy. It is the second most common cause of atraumatic peripheral facial nerve palsy.

15 **Supraorbital Neuralgia** 74

Supraorbital neuralgia is pain in the distribution of the supraorbital nerve that is often caused by a provoking stimulus, such as goggles or helmets. However, other causes should be excluded with history, physical exam and neuroimaging studies.

16 **Glossopharngeal Neuralgia** 79

Glossopharyngeal neuralgia (ninth cranial nerve) presents with severe, brief, stabbing, recurrent pain in the back of the throat and tongue, the tonsils, and part of the ear. Secondary causes must be excluded and treatment focuses on polypharmacy.

17 **Arachnoiditis** 83

The debilitating pain of arachnoiditis can be difficult to treat and progressive. This chapter reviews the causes, sign and symptoms, diagnostic criteria and treatment options available for these patients.

18 Occipital Neuralgia 89

Occipital neuralgia is defined by the International Headache Society (IHS) as paroxysmal shooting or stabbing pain in the dermatomes of the nervus occipitalis major or nervus occipitalis minor. The pain in occipital neuralgia is characterized as burning, lancenating pain that, like migraine, is usually unilateral with radiation to the frontal, orbital and periorbital regions. Treatment flow guidelines start with; history and physical exam, followed by performing a test block, then considering more long-term blocks with anesthetic and corticosteroid or with radiofrequency ablation of the occipital nerve.

19 Cancer Pain 94

With over 10 million cancer survivors in the United States and the incidence of cancer treatment related pain syndromes soaring higher each year, the tumor itself is less often the cause of pain than is the treatment. Knowledge of injuries that can occur due to chemotherapy, surgery and radiation therapy are crucial in trying to understand and manage cancer pain.

20 Mononeuropathy 98

Mononeuropathies are a not uncommon source of pain, of which, one of the most notable is post-herpetic neuralgia, which is covered in its own section of this book. Other notable painful mononeuropathies include, diabetic mononeuropathy and amyotrophy, mononeuropathy multiplex, entrapment neuropathies, and mononeuropathies due to peripheral nerve tumors.

SECTION II CHRONIC PAIN AND RELATED DISORDERS

21 Chronic Pain and Depression 105

In treating patients with chronic pain with a co-morbidity of depression, the focus is on a multimodal approach to their treatment. This chapter reviews the pathophysiology and treatment strategies for patients suffering from chronic pain and depression.

22 Chronic Pain and Addictive Disorder 109

The intersection of pain and addiction to opioids is a problem that has defied understanding and solution since 3000 BCE. While addictive disorders do not make treatment with opioids impossible, they certainly make it more dangerous for our patients and society not to mention the emotional and temporal strain they may place on providers.

23 **Chronic Pain And Other Psychiatric Disorders** 113

Chronic pain patients often present with a co-morbid psychiatric abnormality, of which the anxiety disorders and depression are the most common. Concomittant treatment of the psychiatric disorder not only improves emotional health, but can also improve pain scores, functional improvement, and overall sense of well-being. Treatment with anti-depressants and with psychiatric therapy is the mainstay of treatment.

24 **The Difficult Chronic Pain Patient** 119

The prevalence of Cluster B personality disorders in chronic pain patients may exceed the prevalence in clients seen by parole officers. These patients can be labor intensive, produce feelings of incompetence, can be unfulfilling to care for and may in fact at times be dangerous.

SECTION III TREATMENT OVERVIEW

25 **Antidepressants** 125

Antidepressants are often used for the treatment of chronic pain. This chapter will address the efficacy and indications for their use, as well as a discussion of the classes, adverse effects and their use in clinical practice.

26 **Anticonvulsants** 131

Anticonvulsants are often used for the treatment of chronic pain. This chapter will address the mechanism of action and efficacy of these agents. In addition, indications for their use, adverse effects and their use in clinical practice.

27 **Opioids** 138

With limited evidence documenting efficacy and with serious side-effects that are becoming more apparent every year, the controversy surrounding the use of opioids for non-terminal chronic pain has never been so strident. Risk assessment and monitoring are essential in order to ensure both safety for our patients and society and ensuring our patients access to these drugs which can in select patients be so useful.

28 **Other Adjuvant Drugs** 143

Adjuvant drugs are often used for the treatment of chronic pain. This chapter will address commonly used agents and their use in clinical practice.

29 **Spinal Cord Stimulation and Peripheral Nerve Stimulation** 148

Spinal cord and peripheral nerve stimulation is being used more frequently in chronic pain conditions. This chapter discusses the pathophysiology, indications, surgical procedure, risks and outcomes for patients who utilize these modalities for pain control.

30 **Neurosurgical Procedures for Pain**   155

Neurosurgical techniques have long been used for the treatment of intractable pain. They have been considered the most logical treatment choice for pain in that they would cause a blockade of a patient's pain pathways and thus prevent the transmission of pain signals to the cortex. Over time, neurosurgical techniques have become more sophisticated and there are now multiple modalities being used to treat similar pain states. When determining whether or not neurosurgical intervention is warranted for a patient with intractable pain, many authors have offered that clinicians can pose themselves the question as to the nature of their patient's pain- intractability and quality of pain.

31 **Medical Cannabis**   163

Fifteen States in the US and many countries in the world now permit the use of marijuana as a treatment for chronic pain. There is an expanding body of knowledge endorsing the efficacy of the drug but limited and disputed data surrounding safety. Patients will be asking their providers to help them make decisions regarding the use of marijuana for chronic pain and they must understand the issues.

Index   169

Chronic Pain Conditions

1   Complex Regional Pain Syndrome

A 31-year-old woman presents with a chief complaint of severe pain in her entire right arm. She was in her usual state of good health until 6 months ago, when, while working as a nurse carrying a small bundle of metal-covered charts, her hand came in contact with a counter and her fingers were crushed between the metal charts that she was carrying and the countertop. The total weight of the charts may have been 3 pounds. She developed pain over the proximal phalanges of the first, second, and third fingers, which seemed to become more intense on a daily basis.

The pain over the course of the next two months spread to involve the entirety of her hand and arm up to the proximal humeral region. The distribution was not in the distribution of any peripheral nerve or nerves. The pain was severe and incapacitating. Clothing rubbing on her arm was extremely painful, and when she showered she had to keep that extremity out of the water because it was so painful. She felt that the arm was weak. She noticed that it was reddish in color compared to her other arm, and it felt warm. She also noted a mild tremor in the arm.

When asked about her mood, she stated that she was frustrated and frightened. She has not been able to return to work since the injury, and her orthopedic surgeon, whom she saw for an evaluation, told her that she had reflex sympathetic dystrophy. She was tearful in the office, protective of her arm, and holding it in an extended and dystrophic posture. She felt she was starting to have pain now on the left as well, also in the proximal phalanges of the first, second, and third fingers.

She was using 10 mg of amitriptyline at bedtime and ibuprofen 800 mg q4h without any noticeable relief.

What do you do now?

This patient is likely suffering from complex regional pain syndrome. The vast majority of the literature surrounding complex regional pain syndrome has been published following wars. The first report was written following the Civil War and described a brachial plexus projectile injury. Since then, there have been approximately 50 names applied to the same disorder, including reflex sympathetic dystrophy (RSD), causalgia, foot and hand syndrome, and so forth. Current nomenclature attempts to place all of these diseases under the same heading, and that proper heading is complex regional pain syndrome (CRPS). Reflex sympathetic dystrophy nomenclature is applied only to a limited degree, in describing Type 1 CRPS, because it has been shown that this disorder is not exclusively a disorder of the sympathetic nervous system; it does not typically involve dystrophy; and it is not a reflex. It is, however, complex; it is usually regional, usually affects an extremity, and it is a pain syndrome.

DIAGNOSTIC CRITERIA

In current nomenclature CRPS Type 1 (RSD) describes a disorder that does not involve injury to a major nerve. CRPS Type 2 (causalgia) describes an identical disorder, but with injury to a major nerve. The injury to the major nerve is the only distinguishing criterion between Type 1 and Type 2. Sensitivity and specificity of most defining diagnostic criteria (e.g., International Association for the Study of Pain) used for establishing a diagnosis remains 98% and 38%, respectively. This means that using the usual standard criteria for diagnosis, you will rarely ever miss a diagnosis but you will only be correct in making the diagnosis 38% of the time. Thus, CRPS is very frequently overdiagnosed.

Modifications in the criteria have been described, changing sensitivity to 70% and specificity to 95%. These criteria for diagnosis include the following:

1. There is no other diagnosis that can account for the patient's symptoms and signs.
2. There is pain out of proportion to the injury.
3. Signs and symptoms are present in the following categories (see Figure 1.1):

   a. Motor.
   The symptom would be the fact that the patient describes a sensation of weakness.

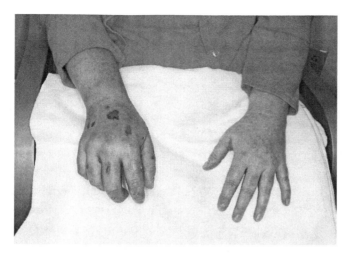

FIGURE 1.1 Vasomotor and sudomotor dysfunction and edema in a patient with CPRS of the right upper extremity. (Courtesy of Gilbert J. Fanciullo, MD, MS, Department of Anesthesiology, Section of Pain Medicine, Dartmouth Hitchcock Medical Center, Lebanon, NH.)

The sign would be that on physical examination there is weakness identified.

b. Vasomotor.
The symptom would be that the patient describes temperature or color changes.
The sign would be that the examiner observes color changes and measures temperature changes.

c. Sudomotor/Edema.
The symptom would be that the patient describes swelling or increased sweating in the affected extremity.
The sign would be that swelling is noted by an examiner and increased moisture is objectively noted by the examiner as well.

d. Sensory.
The symptom would be that the patient describes pain in the affected extremity.
The sign would be the presence of allodynia, hyperalgesia, or hyperpathia.

In order to meet criteria for a diagnosis, a patient would have to have symptoms in all four categories and signs in two of the four categories. The specificity of the diagnosis increases if there are signs in three categories, and increases again if there are signs in four categories.

There also exists good data on "spreading" of the affected area in CRPS. The spreading is not part of the criteria most examiners use; however, it is extremely rare to encounter CRPS patients who have not had spreading of their disorder. The spreading may occur continuously (as in the patient described above), where the injury, which often occurs as the result of a trivial mechanism, begins in a distal portion of the extremity and spreads to involve the entirety of that extremity. The spreading may also occur in a mirror-image fashion, also present in the patient presented, such that the pain began in one hand and the patient would start to experience pain in the identical area in the other hand, or it may involve spreading to an entirely different extremity. The patient will often state that the symptoms feel identical to the symptoms in the original extremity. There are case reports of total body complex regional pain syndrome, but many experienced clinicians question this disorder. There is frequently psychopathology noted in patients presenting with CRPS, but this is not different from patients presenting with any severe, painful disorder.

Radiological changes had been described early in the 20th century and three-phase bone scintography had been suggested and commonly used as a diagnostic tool. It has subsequently been shown that almost half of patients with CRPS have a normal bone scan.

Three distinct stages were described in the early 1950s:

- Stage I was characterized by pain and sensory abnormalities, vasomotor and sudomotor dysfunction, and edema.
- Stage II (dystrophic stage) occurred 3–6 months after onset and was described as having more pain and sensory dysfunction plus development of significant motor and trophic changes.
- Stage III was thought to be distinguished by decreased pain and increased motor and trophic changes.

Researchers have conducted elegant studies ultimately employing cluster analysis to determine if patients with different symptom complexes as described above can be sorted by duration of symptoms. Their results, as well as empirical work of others, argue against sequential stages of CRPS.

Three possible CRPS subtypes have been described and include:

- Limited syndrome with vasomotor signs predominating
- Limited syndrome with neuropathic pain/sensory abnormalities predominating
- Florid CRPS syndrome similar to "classic RSD" descriptions

MANAGEMENT

Nonpharmacologic Treatment

Treatment is often labor intensive and unsuccessful. Only one in five patients diagnosed with CRPS will be able to continue to work. It is generally believed that physical medicine treatments are the most important part of treatment of CRPS, and that any other remedy should be directed toward enabling the patient to have physical therapy and to remain active. There is little evidence to support this contention.

Treatment is directed along four vectors. The first is physical medicine, and despite the lack of evidence supporting the exclusivity of usefulness of this intervention, it is certainly extremely important and should be provided for any patient diagnosed with complex regional pain syndrome. The second vector is behavioral medicine. These patients often have severe and unrelenting pain that is refractory to treatment. Depression and anxiety are highly prevalent in this population and should be treated; and behavioral approaches to managing the pain should be implemented immediately upon diagnosis. The third vector is pharmacologic treatment, and the fourth is procedural and surgical treatment.

Pharmacologic Treatment

From a pharmacological perspective, nonsteroidal anti-inflammatory drugs, antidepressants, and anticonvulsants should be implemented aggressively, and the disorder should be treated pharmacologically as a neuropathic pain syndrome. Gabapentin with a target dose of 3600 mg per day or pregabalin with a target dose of 450 mg per day, duloxetine with a target dose of 60 mg per day, or another mixed-type antidepressant should be instituted. The vast majority of these patients will require treatment with opioids as well. General rules regarding opioids should be followed, and there may be (as with all neuropathic pain syndromes) an advantage to selecting methadone as the opioid of choice because of its NMDA receptor antagonist properties.

The use of ketamine infusions or intranasal ketamine appears to be a very promising avenue for treatment and there is an expanding body of literature supporting this modality. It should be considered and instituted as quickly as possible after diagnosis.

Procedural and Surgical Treatment

These patients should also be offered sympathetic blockade as soon as possible after diagnosis. Despite the severance of the strict tie between the sympathetic nervous system and CRPS, pain in CRPS can be sympathetically maintained and sympathetic blocks can often provide a reduction in pain for some period of time. Rarely will CRPS be cured by sympathetic blockade. It is recommended that physical therapy appointments should follow the sympathetic procedures by a brief number of hours in order to enable physical therapy. In the case of upper-extremity CRPS, stellate ganglion blocks are the sympathetic blockade treatment of choice, as lumbar sympathetic blocks are for the lower extremities. In rare cases, an epidural catheter can be implanted and the patient can be admitted to the hospital for intensive pain relief and physical therapy.

The above-mentioned treatments should be initiated simultaneously and aggressively in order to try to get the patient's pain under control. If the patient's pain is not quickly brought into a reasonable realm, then the patient should be considered for a trial and possible implantation of a spinal cord stimulating device. Spinal cord stimulators have been shown to be extremely effective in patients with CRPS and, unless there is a dramatic response to other treatments, this treatment should be implemented as soon as possible in order to prevent spreading, relieve pain, reduce psychopathology, improve function, and hopefully to return the patient to their previous level of function.

CONCLUSION

Eighty percent of patients with CRPS are never able to return to work. It is a disorder that requires intensive and long-term management. It is best accomplished in a multidisciplinary way and care should include physicians, mental health specialists, and physical medicine specialists.

- Complex regional pain syndrome is often overdiagnosed, and strict criteria should be used to make the diagnosis.
- Treatment should be aggressive, multimodal, and multidisciplinary.
- The use of ketamine and spinal cord stimulation should be considered early in the treatment paradigm to prevent spreading and disability.

Further Reading

Allen G, Galer BS, Schwartz L. Epidemiology of complex regional pain syndrome: a retrospective chart review of 134 patients. *Pain* 1999;80:539-544.

Bonica JJ. *The Management of Pain*. Kimpton, London, 1953.

Bruehl S, Harden RN, Galer BS, et al. External validation of IASP diagnostic criteria for Complex Regional Pain Syndrome and proposed research diagnostic criteria. *Pain* 1999;81:147-154.

Bruehl S, Harden RN, Galer BS, et al. Complex regional pain syndrome: are there distinct subtypes and sequential stages of the syndrome? *Pain* 2002;95:119-124.

Evans JA. Reflex sympathetic dystrophy. *Surg Clin North Am* 1946;26:780-790.

Harden RN. A clinical approach to complex regional pain syndrome. *Clin J Pain* 2000;16:S26-S32.

Livingstone WK. Posttraumatic pain syndromes. *West J Surg Obst Gynec* 1938;46:341-347.

Mitchell SW. *Injuries of Nerves and Their Consequences*. Lippincott, Philadelphia, 1874.

Mitchell SW, Moorehouse GR, Keene WW. *Gunshot Wounds and Other Injuries of Nerves*. Lippincott, Philadelphia, 1864.

Perez RSGM, Kwakkel G, Zuurmond WWA, de Lange JJ. Treatment of reflex sympathetic dystrophy (CRPS Type I): a research synthesis of 21 randomized trials. *J Pain Sympt Manage* 2001;21(6):511-526.

Raja SN, Grabow TS. Complex regional pain syndrome I (reflex sympathetic dystrophy) *Anesthesiology* 2002;96:1254-1260.

Rommel O, Malin J, Zenz M, Janig W. Quantitative sensory testing, neurophysiological and psychological examination in patients with complex regional pain syndrome and hemisensory deficits. *Pain* 2001;93:279-293.

Stanton-Hicks M, Janig W, Hassenbusch S, et al. Reflex sympathetic dystrophy: changing concepts and taxonomy. *Pain* 1995;63:127-133.

Wilson PR, Stanton-Hicks M, Harden RN, *CRPS: Current Diagnosis and Therapy*. Progress in Pain Research and Management, Volume 32. IASP Press, Seattle, 2005. Excellent and useful review.

2 Peripheral Neuropathy

A 55-year-old man with a 10-year history of type II diabetes presents to your clinic with bilateral lower-extremity pain. Approximately one year ago, he noticed burning and tingling in his feet that has subsequently begun to interfere with his daily activities and social interactions. He used to work full-time at an office job; however, secondary to pain, he presently is working part-time. He has noticed that walking has become more of a chore, although he denies any gait instability or falls.

His pain is described as sharp, shooting, and burning pain, which is worse at the end of the day when he takes his shoes off or settles down at night. In addition, he awakens at night because of severe pain in his feet and sometimes into his legs. He denies any numbness or weakness. His primary care physician (PCP) has prescribed the tricyclic antidepressant desipramine to manage his pain, but the patient did not respond adequately and experienced dizziness and constipation. His PCP has referred him to a pain specialist for further evaluation and treatment.

He denies any chest pain or shortness of breath. He denies any other symptoms and has had no fever, chills, cough, bloody stools, or hematuria. His physical examination was normal except for hyperesthesia of both feet as well as decreased vibratory sensation. A review of his labs revealed his hemoglobin A1c was 8.0% (normal less than 6%). His remaining labs were read as normal.

He had been referred to Neurology, EMG was read as normal, and based on the physical exam findings and history patient was diagnosed with diabetic peripheral neuropathy. The patient presents to the Pain Clinic for further management of his pain.

What do you do now?

This patient is likely suffering from diabetic peripheral neuropathic pain. The patient's pain is not adequately controlled and he has had side effects to the tricyclic antidepressants (TCAs) that were prescribed by his primary care physician. His continued pain is affecting his quality of life and he requires further pain control.

DIAGNOSTIC CRITERIA

The initial step, as always, is to confirm the diagnosis of diabetic peripheral neuropathic pain. The practitioner can rely on patients' subjective description and physical examination findings to diagnose neuropathic pain. Moresophisticated tests include electromyography and nerve conduction velocity, which were performed in this particular patient. Interpretations of these tests have certain limitations, as negative results do not rule out the possible diagnosis of neuropathy, because the tests do not detect changes in small nerve fibers, which can be affected in peripheral neuropathy.

It is also important to eliminate other potential serious conditions, as in the Rochester Diabetic Neuropathic Study, where approximately 10% of patients with diabetes had symptoms attributable to nondiabetic causes. There is a wide array of causes for polyneuropathies, and diabetes is only one cause (Table 2.1). Many of the diagnoses can be excluded through a careful history, such as neuropathies based on exposure or familial neuropathies based on family history.

Patients with neuropathic pain often describe allodynia, dysesthesia, hyperalgesia, hyperpathia, and paresthesias, therefore subjective evaluation is helpful in diagnosis (see Table 2.2).

A complete physical exam is important to assess vibration, light touch, temperature, sensation, reflexes, and proprioception. Laboratory studies should include a complete blood count, general chemistries, evaluation of hemoglobin A1c, TSH to rule out thyroid disease, B12 and folate to measure for pernicious anemia. If suspicion regarding etiology still exists, other testing such antinuclear antibody, sedimentation rate, rheumatoid factor, and urine protein electrophoresis might be appropriate (see Table 2.3).

Nerve conduction studies may help to pinpoint specific diagnosis. Electromyography can distinguish between weakness from a nerve or a muscle disorder. Nerve biopsy for patients with severe and progressive

TABLE 2.1 **Differential Diagnoses of Symmetric Polyneuropathies**

Type	Syndrome
Congenital/familial	Charcot-Marie-Tooth, amyloid neuropathy, Fabry disease.
Traumatic	Entrapment syndromes.
Inflammatory/infiltrative	Sarcoidosis, leprosy, Lyme disease, HIV, amyloidosis, periarteritis nodosa.
Neoplastic	Carcinoma, paraneoplastic syndrome, myeloma, leukemias, lymphomas.
Metabolic/endocrine	Diabetes, uremia, pernicious anemia, hypothyroidism, acute, intermittent porphyria.
Vascular	Diabetes, vasculitis
Toxic	Alcohol, heavy metals (lead, mercury, arsenic), hydrocarbon, chemotherapeutics, and drugs (pyridoxine), isoniazid, antiretrovirals.
Autoimmune	Diabetes, phospholipid antibody syndrome, chronic, inflammatory, demyelinating polyneuropathy (CIDP), multifocal motor neuropathy, Guillain-Barré syndrome.

Adapted from Green DA, Pfeifer MA, Oletsky JM, Shervin RS, eds. *Diabetes Management and Complications*. Churchill, Livingston, New York, 1985. Vinik A. Diagnosis and management of diabetic neuropathy. *Clin Geriater Med* 1999;15:293-315.

disease can identify vasculitis, amyloidosis, sarcoidosis, and other hereditary neuropathies.

MANAGEMENT

Depending on the etiology of the peripheral neuropathic pain, the treatment is often focused on the underlying etiology, as well as symptomatic management. Chronic pain is a lifelong dynamic process and neuropathy cannot be reversed; therefore, pain management will be an important component to treatment for the entirety of the patient's life.

TABLE 2.2 **Symptoms and Definitions**

Symptom	Definition
Allodynia	Pain from stimuli that are not normally painful.
Dysesthesia	Unpleasant, abnormal sensation which may be associated with a burning, shooting, or electric sensation; may be spontaneous or touch evoked.
Hyperalgesia	Exaggerated response to a stimulus that is normally painful.
Hyperpathia	Painful, increased reaction to a stimulus.
Paresthesias	Abnormal, non-painful sensation which may involve weakness or loss of sensation.

If the underlying etiology is diabetic peripheral neuropathy (DPN), improved glycemic control will not reverse the damage; however, it may prevent further neuropathic damage. If any other etiology is discovered, such as a vitamin B12 deficiency, treatment should be geared toward stabilizing B12 levels.

The goal of any pain management plan is to reduce the intensity of pain. It is important for the clinician to inform the patient that although treatment can reduce their pain level, it does not generally eliminate pain completely. The clinician should be vigilant for signs of comorbid psychiatric conditions, most notably depression, anxiety, and sleep dysfunction. Studies have found that 70% of patients with chronic pain have sleep disturbances, and between 22% and 78% are depressed. These interrelationships can exacerbate pain, and therefore need to be part of a patient's pain treatment.

TABLE 2.3 **Initial Assessment of Pain**

1. Review past medical records and diagnostic studies.
2. Obtain a detailed history including pain characteristic and intensity.
3. Conduct a thorough physical exam.
4. Obtain a thorough psychosocial assessment including sleep disturbance, work-related issues, and availability of family support.
5. Provide an appropriate diagnostic workup to determine the cause of pain.

Dworkin RH, Backonja M, Rowbotham MC, et al. Advances in neuropathic pain: diagnosis, mechanisms, and treatment recommendations. *Arch Neurol* 2003;60:1524-1534.

Patients should also be counseled on the importance of daily examinations of their feet for early signs of ulcers, and should receive information about proper footwear.

Pharmacologic Treatment

Evidence-based therapy for the treatment of DPN should be instituted for pain management (see Table 2.4). There are several different classes of drugs in the management of peripheral neuropathy; these include serotonin norepinephrine reuptake inhibitors (SNRIs), TCAs, alpha2-delta ligands, anticonvulsants, opioids, and topical agents. Currently, duloxetine (SNRI) and pregabalin (anticonvulsant) are approved by the FDA for the management of neuropathic pain associated with DPN. Although opioids are approved for the management of moderate to severe pain, they are also used at times in the management of pain associated with peripheral neuropathy. Combining medications from these categories helps some patients for whom monotherapy has failed. It is important to note that treatment for this condition is limited by side effects and medication interactions, especially in the elderly or in patients with severe, comorbid conditions.

TABLE 2.4 **Pharmacologic Treatment of Diabetic Peripheral Neuropathy**

Medication	Typical Effective Dosage
SNRIs (serotonin norepinephrine reuptake inhibitors) Duloxetine, venlafaxine	See chapter 25
Tricyclic Antidepressants Amitriptyline, desipramine, nortriptyline	See chapter 25
Anticonvulsants Gabapentin, pregabalin, lamotrigine, valproate, topiramate	See chapter 26
Opioids tramadol, oxycodone, morphine, methadone	See chapter 27
Topical Agents Lidocaine, compounding agent	See chapter 28

Procedural and Surgical Treatment

Procedural therapy—including lumbar sympathetic blocks, intrathecal pumps, or epidural catheters—is not a common practice, as there is little evidence that these benefit patients with peripheral neuropathies.

However, although interventional techniques have not been shown to be effective for the majority of patients who have diabetic peripheral neuropathy, some patients may benefit from injections, neurostimulatory approaches, and neuraxial approaches.

KEY POINTS TO REMEMBER

- Diabetic peripheral neuropathy is a diagnosis of exclusion. The clinician should focus on a detailed history, review of systems, physical exam, and appropriate lab tests to rule out other potential causes.
- The underlying etiology should be treated.
- Medical treatment of diabetic peripheral neuropathy is usually successful with polytherapy.
- It is also important to treat patients' psychiatric comorbidities, as this will help to control their pain.

Further Reading

Argoff CE. The coexistence of neuropathic pain, sleep, and psychiatric disorders: a novel treatment approach. *Clin J Pain* 2007;23:15-22.

Argoff CE, Backonja MM, Belgrade NJ, et al. Consensus guidelines: treatment planning and options. *Mayo Clin Proc* 2006;81(4 Suppl):S12-S25.

Boucek P, Advanced diabetic neuropathy: a point of no return? *Rev Diabet Stud* 2006;3:143-150.

Duloxetine Hydrochloride (package insert). Indianapolis, IN: Eli Lily and Company; 2007.

Pregabalin (package insert). Vega Baha, PR: Pfizer Pharmaceuticals Loc; 2007.

3 Postherpetic Neuralgia

A 74-year-old man presented to the emergency department 2 months prior with a painful rash on his right buttock and leg. He was subsequently diagnosed with herpes zoster and was placed on prednisone and valacyclovir. In spite of treatment, the patient developed severe, neuropathic pain in his right lower extremity and was placed on oxycodone.

He describes burning and aching pain located in his right buttock radiating down the posterolateral aspect of his thigh into his calf and into the plantar surface of his foot. His pain is so severe that it causes tremors. It is episodic, daily pain lasting minutes.

His pain continued despite oxycodone, and so his primary care physician placed him on hydromorphone and amitriptyline, without substantial benefit. When he presents to the Pain Clinic, his pain is so severe that he requires a wheelchair for ambulation.

His past medical history is significant for gout, gastroesophageal reflux disease, prostate cancer status post radiation therapy, and shingles. His review of systems is positive for weight loss secondary to pain, hearing loss, urinary incontinence and burning, sleep dysfunction, and pain. His physical exam findings are positive for a rash with healing lesions in the right buttock extending down the posterior aspect of his leg, knee, and into his calf. He also has allodynia and dysesthesia in the same distribution with multiple scabs; no ulcerations, vesicles, or drainage. He presents to the Pain Clinic for intractable pain related to postherpetic neuralgia in the distribution of L5-S1 on the right.

What do you do now?

EPIDEMIOLOGY

Shingles (herpes zoster) and its chronic, painful sequela, postherpetic neuralgia (PHN), is the most common neuropathic disease affecting 20% of the American population who have otherwise been healthy. Reactivation of the virus occurs and is spread corresponding to the sensory dermatome.

Herpes zoster (HZ) is a focal resurgence of the varicella zoster virus that has been dormant in the sensory ganglia since an episode of chickenpox (varicella) acquired during childhood. HZ is a common disease with a reported incidence of up to 3.4 per 100,000 patients per year. The most common location is thoracic followed by the first trigeminal division of the upper face. However, shingles and subsequently PHN can affect any area of the body. Risk factors for herpes zoster include age when immunocompetence declines and immunosuppression from disease or medications (corticosteroids); however, the majority of shingles occurs in otherwise healthy, older individuals.

DIAGNOSTIC CRITERIA

Diagnosis of PHN is based on a history of previous zoster in the same dermatome as the chronic pain and could include physical exam findings of persistent scars. This diagnosis can be challenging, however, if the rash is subtle or not noticed by either the patient or the physician (zoster without rash). If there is a question about the diagnosis, further workup should be performed to exclude another etiology, such as radiologic studies to evaluate for nerve compression by a tumor or spinal pathology.

SIGNS AND SYMPTOMS

Patients with PHN can experience tactile or mechanical allodynia, and will often avoid contact of the affected skin with clothing, bed sheets, or even a light breeze. Other patients complain of hyperalgesia or exaggerated pain following a minimally painful stimulus. A minority of patients also complain of lancinating pains, which are brief jolts of severe pain. Motor symptoms are not a usual component, as the zoster virus affects the sensory nerves only, however, patients with shingles can develop weakness secondary to disuse, and loss of deep tendon reflexes. In rare cases, patients can have visceral involvement or neurogenic bladder or rectum.

MANAGEMENT

Nonpharmacologic Treatment

Nonpharmacologic treatments for PHN are of little benefit, as the recovery appears to be regeneration of damaged axons, and this has not been shown to be influenced by nonpharmacologic treatment. However, they can be beneficial for the treatment of problems associated with PHN including inactivity and depression.

In regard to procedural therapy, there is little evidence that epidurals have been beneficial, and these are usually instituted if pharmacologic treatment is ineffective. Epidurals have been slightly efficacious in early PHN, and injections of local steroids at the area of scars that may be involved in the increased pain have not shown to decrease pain.

Nerve or spinal cord stimulators (see chapter 29) have been proven effective for treating other types of neuropathic pain; unfortunately, there are few studies in PHN.

Pharmacologic Treatment

Immediate treatment of shingles with antiviral medications, and tricyclic antidepressants has been shown to lessen the likelihood and severity of PHN. Treatment of established PHN is similar to treatment for other neuropathic pain syndromes, with medications as the most effective therapeutic options for these patients. There have been four classes of medications that have documented efficacy and safety in placebo-controlled, double-blind studies for PHN:

1. Topical local anesthetics (see chapter 28) act locally, making them ideal for patients because of minimal risk of side effects and drug interactions.
   a. The Lidoderm Patch® contains 5% lidocaine and is FDA approved for PHN.
   b. Topical creams and ointments containing capsaicin, the substance found in chili peppers, are not widely used because of the intolerable side effects of burning sensation when applied.

c. There have been a few, small, clinical trials of topical, nonsteroidal anti-inflammatory drugs (NSAIDs) that have been conducted with uneven results.

2. Tricyclic antidepressants (TCA) (see chapter 25) are commonly used for treating PHN and other types of neuropathic pain. The TCAs have been effective for persistent, ongoing, lancinating pain, and allodynia. However, there are a multitude of side effects to TCAs including cognitive changes, constipation, dry eyes and mouth, orthostatic hypotension and sexual dysfunction. Narrow-angle glaucoma and cardiac dysrhythmia are relative contraindications to using TCAs. They are not a first-line treatment option for the elderly and are listed as contraindicated for use in patients who are older than 65 by the American Geriatric Society. Amitriptyline has serotinergic as well as adrenergic potentiation in comparison to the secondary adrenergic-specific amines, nortriptyline or desipramine. Thus, amitriptyline has a more specific side-effect profile that is often intolerable for patients.

3. Anticonvulsants (see chapter 26) decrease neuronal hyperexcitability making them often efficacious for patients with herpetic neuropathic pain.

a. Gabapentin has been well evaluated for PHN in multicenter, randomized, controlled trials. Gabapentin has minimal drug-drug interactions, and serious side effects are rare; however, the most common side effects include sedation, cognitive dysfunction, and peripheral edema. Gabapentin is renally excreted, and doses may need to be decreased in patients with poor creatinine clearance.

b. Second-line treatments for PHN include carbamazepine, which is FDA approved for the treatment of neuralgia and phenytoin.

4. Opioids (see chapter 27) have been shown effective and safe for PHN in several double-blind and placebo-controlled studies. Risk of abuse is particularly low among the elderly population unless there is a prior history. Opioids are often a first-line treatment option for geriatric patients, and the extended release are preferable for chronic pain; however, shorter-acting

agents may have fewer side effects and may result in less accumulation of metabolites in the older patients.

It is difficult to predict which patients will respond to which medications, and it is often necessary to try several medications and to establish polymedication therapy for optimal treatment. Elderly patients should be treated with attention to cognitive dysfunction, hypotension, constipation, urinary retention, and cardiac arrhythmias when prescribing these medications.

These four classes of medications have documented efficacy and safety for postherpetic neuralgia, as described previously. No single treatment surpasses the other, and consideration of these treatments should be based on patients' symptoms, age, comorbidities, and medication history.

KEY POINTS TO REMEMBER

- Postherpetic neuralgia is a devastating consequence of shingles (herpes zoster).
- The elderly and the immunocompromised are at higher risk of developing PHN.
- Four classes of medications are documented in clinical trials to be effective and safe, and these include topical local anesthetics, tricyclic antidepressants, anticonvulsants, and opioids.
- Elderly patients should be treated with attention to potential side effects of treatment.

Further Reading

AGS Panel on Chronic Pain in Older Persons. The management of chronic pain in older persons: AGS Panel on Chronic Pain in Older Persons. American Geriatric Society. *J Am Geriatr Fsc* 1998;46:635-651.

Bowsher D. Acute herpes zoster post-herpetic neuralgia: acyclovir and now treatment with amitriptyline. *Br J Gen Pract* 1992; 42:244-246.

Chadda VS, Mathur MS. Double-blind study of the effects of diphenylhydantoin sodium on diabetic neuropathy. *J Assoc Physicians India* 1978;26:403-406.

Donohue JG, Choo PW, Manson JE, Platt R. The incidence of herpes zoster. *Arch Intern Med* 1995;155:11605-11609.

Galer BS, Jensen MP, Ma T, Davies PS, Rowbotham MC. Lidocaine Patch® five percent effectively treats all neuropathic pain qualities: results in a randomized, double-blinded, vehicle-controlled, three-week efficacy study with the use of the neuropathic pain scale. *Clin J Pain* 2002;18:297-301.

Gerson GR, Jones RB, Luscomb DK. Studies on the concomitant use of carbamazepine and clomipramine for the relief of post-herpetic neuralgia. *Post-Grad Med J* 1977;53(Suppl 4):104-109.

Gilden DH, Duland AN, Devlin ME, Mahalingam R, Cohrs R. Varicella-zoster virus reactivation without rash. *J Infect Dos* 1992;166(Suppl 1):S30-S34.

Harke H, Gretenkort P, Ladleif HU, Koster P, Rahman S. Spinal cord stimulation in post-herpetic neuralgia and acute herpes zoster pain. *Anesth Analg* 2002; 94:694-700.

Hoop-Simpson, RE. Post-herpetic neuralgia. *J R Coll Gen Pract* 1975;25:571-575.

Kost RG, Straus SE, Post-herpetic neuralgia: pathogenesis, treatment and prevention. *N Engl J Med* 1996;335:32-42.

Rice AS, Maton S. Gabapentin in post-herpetic neuralgia: a randomized, double-blind, placebo-controlled study. *Pain* 2001;94:215-224.

Rowbotham MC, Harden N, Stacey B, Bernstein P, Magnus-Miller L. Gabapentin for the treatment of post-herpetic neuralgia: a randomized, controlled trial. *JAMA* 1998;280:1837-1842.

Watson CP, Babul N. Efficacy of oxycodone on neuropathic pain: a randomized trial on post-herpetic neuralgia. *Neurology* 1998;50:1837-1848.

Watson CPN, Evans RJ, Reed K, Mersky H, Goldsmith L, Warsh J. Amitriptyline versus placebo in post-herpetic neuralgia. *Neurology* 1992;32:671-673.

Watson CPN, Evans RJ, Watt BR, Birkett N. Post-herpetic neuralgia: 208 cases. *Pain* 1988;35:289-297.

Watson CPN, Vernich L, Chipman M, Reed K. Nortriptyline versus amitriptyline in post-herpetic neuralgia: a randomized trial. *Neurology* 1998;51:1166-1171.

4 Central Post-Stroke Pain

A 45-year-old female presents to the clinic after suffering a left-sided brainstem infarct, with signs and symptoms of a partial Wallenberg syndrome. Computerized tomography and magnetic resonance imaging show a left lateral medullary infarct. A painful condition on her right side developed ten days after the initial stroke. Symptoms included numbness of the left face and in the right thoracic and abdominal areas. She also experienced tingling in the right arm. In the right leg, she complained of tingling, aching pain that is continuous in nature and burning pain when she has close contact with any fabric or breeze on her leg, as well as being worse in cold weather, but improved in warm weather. She rates her pain as a 4-9/10 in severity and continuous in nature. She denies any weakness of her arms, legs, or face. She was reevaluated 6 months later and was found to have similar symptoms of pain in her right leg. Given the quality of her pain and her recent stroke, she was diagnosed with central post-stroke pain.

What do you do now?

This patient's diagnosis is central post-stroke pain (CPSP). CPSP is an often underdiagnosed and frequently overlooked disorder. Often considered only in association with thalamic pain syndrome following infarct to the thalamus, pain following stroke may occur with any setting of stroke affecting nociceptive pain fibers at any level. Neuropathic or central pain can occur in up to 8% of patients after a stroke. Multiple hypotheses have been offered as to the etiology of the pain, of which the most commonly accepted is that damage occurs in the spinothalamocortical sensory pathways. Pain onset can occur within 1 month in 63%, between 1 and 6 months in 19%, and after 6 months in 19% of patients.

SIGNS AND SYMPTOMS

The diagnosis of CPSP is considered in the setting of pain following ischemic or hemorrhagic stroke, with either positive or negative sensory symptoms in the same distribution:

- Negative symptoms include numbness.
- Positive symptoms include burning, tingling, sharp, and lancinating pain.

The pain associated with CPSP may be spontaneous or evoked. The evoked pain can be brought on by both nociceptive and non-nociceptive stimuli. CPSP patients usually describe their pain as aching, pricking, lancinating, shooting, squeezing, and throbbing either in a continuous or in an intermittent fashion. The pain may be worsened with movement, touch, temperature changes—specifically cold temperatures, and by both physical and emotional stress. The intensity of the pain may vary over its course, but can be quite burdensome. Allodynia, hyperalgesia, or dysesthesia may be found at bedside.

Patients with CPSP will most likely have other negative sensory symptoms in a similar distribution including impairment in pinprick, touch, and most commonly, a decrease in temperature sensation. Vibration sense and proprioceptive loss is less frequent, but can occur. The most common distribution is hemibody and contralateral to the stroke, but can occur in any location of the face, arm, or leg even ipsilateral to the stroke lesion. Weakness does not necessarily have to be present, but can occur in up to 60% of patients. The weakness can include hemiplegia, dysmetria, and tremor.

TABLE 4.1 **Secondary Causes of Central Post-Stroke Pain**

Peripheral neuropathy and other neuralgias

Psychological causes

Ulcerations

Deep venous thrombosis

Pericapsulitis

When diagnosing CPSP, other causes of pain should be excluded (Table 4.1).

DIAGNOSTIC CRITERIA

Pain drawings can be highly useful. The drawing can delineate the neuro-anatomical distribution of the patient's pain and sensory deficits.

MRI imaging is most useful specifically for detecting acute stroke events. CT imaging may also be useful; however, clarity of smaller lesions may be more difficult to assess. MRI imaging may show multiple lesions in CPSP patients—many of which may not be pain producing. Ventroposterolateral thalamic lesions are most likely to produce pain; however, lesions anywhere in the sensory pathways may produce pain symptoms. It has been described that lesions found in the post central gyrus tended to not produce CPSP. It also appears that lesions in the insular and opercular regions tend to produce CPSP as these areas appear to play an important role in modulating pain and thermal sensation.

MANAGEMENT

Pharmacologic Treatment

Antidepressants (See Table 25.1)

Amitriptyline was the first drug proven to be effective for the treatment of CPSP. In a double-blind placebo-controlled crossover study, 10 out of 15 patients with CPSP treated with amitriptyline 75 mg showed improvement of their pain at weeks 2 of a 4-week period versus 1 out of 15 patients treated with placebo. Fourteen out of 15 patients treated with amitriptyline reported adverse side effects but there was no drug-related withdrawal from the study. A study exploring the prophylactic efficacy of amitriptyline showed that 21% of 39 patients with thalamic stroke developed CPSP while taking placebo and 17% while receiving prophylactic treatment with amitriptyline up to 75 mg; thus, amitriptyline was not effective in preventing CPSP due to thalamic stroke.

Just as with the treatment of peripheral neuropathic pain, multiple antidepressants have been used to treat CPSP, specifically those antidepressants that act as selective serotonin reuptake inhibitors (SSRIs) and those medications with some adrenergic properties (i.e., tricyclic antidepressants, selective norepinephrine reuptake inhibitors). Fluvoxamine is an SSRI that has been studied in an open label trial of 31 patients with CPSP. Up to 125 mg was used and showed some efficacy, where the average pain score was reduced from 7.7 to 6.0 on a visual analog scale. Its effect was not related to its antidepressant activity and was most useful in those patients who had a stroke within 1 year. Citalopram has been tried in a small number of patients and did not show any effectiveness.

Anticonvulsants (See Table 26.2)

Carbamazepine has been studied in conjunction with the aforementioned open label amitriptyline study. Carbamazepine was minimally effective, in that it was minimally better than placebo only, at the 3-week assessment period. Some specialists recommend carbamazepine be used as add-on therapy in addition to antidepressants, but the efficacy of the combination has not been proven.

Lamotrigine has been proven to be a moderately effective medication for the treatment of CPSP. In a class I randomized double-blind, placebo-controlled, crossover study, Lamotrigine 200 mg per day reduced the median pain score to 5 from 7 with placebo in the intention-to-treat population of 27 patients.

Gabapentin has not proven to be effective for the treatment of CPSP. Phenytoin, zonisamide, and topiramate have been trialed in a small population of patients with CPSP and have not shown any conclusive evidence for their efficacy in treating CPSP.

Anesthetics (See Chapter 28)

Lidocaine was evaluated in a randomized, double-blind, placebo-controlled trial of 16 patients with neuropathic pain, of which 60% had CPSP. Lidocaine at a dose of 5 mg/kg IV over 30 minutes was significantly more effective in improving spontaneous continuous pain up to 45 minutes following the infusion: 62.5% had significant spontaneous pain relief following the infusion. The effect declined to a negligible level by 2–6 hours. Lidocaine was also able to significantly reduce brush allodynia and mechanical hyperalgesia, but this effect was not found to be significantly better than placebo. Three weeks after completion of the first arm of the study, 12 patients were given mexiletine weekly up to 400–800 mg and were reevaluated after 4–12 months: 25% of patient experienced moderate pain relief, 1 patient had slight pain relief, and 8 patients did not have any relief. Thus, mexiletine is not proven to be effective and had a high side-effect profile.

Other anesthetics such as IV propofol and pentothal have been studied and have been shown to be effective for a short period in those with CPSP.

Opioids

The effectiveness of opioids to populations of patients with CPSP and central pain syndromes has consistently yielded disappointing results. Morphine's effect on treatment of continuing pain was not significantly different from placebo and caused significant side effects when used. This was also the case with naloxone and oral levorphanol. Tramodol was tried in 1 patient with CPSP at 50 mg IV over 5 minutes, and then 20 mg of codeine phosphate and 25 mg of milnacepram was given. The patient had complete pain relief for 5 hours and was asymptomatic for 10 months with codeine phosphate and milnacepram. This study was a class IV study and was the only one performed.

NMDA Antagonists

Ketamine and dextromethorphan have both been studied for their effectiveness in treating CPSP. While ketamine has been tried in refractory CPSP patients and shown to have some benefit as a short-term measure, dextromethorphan was not shown to be effective. Ketamine was examined in an uncontrolled trial with a dose of 5 mg every 5 minutes to a total dose of 25 mg. Eleven patients had more than 40% pain relief, which lasted less than one hour.

Procedural and Surgical Treatment

Nonpharmacologic treatment of CPSP has been proposed and studied, including invasive motor cortex stimulation, deep brain stimulation (DBS), repetitive transcranial magnetic stimulation (rTMS), and vestibulocochlear stimulation. Studies to date indicate that motor cortex stimulation should be considered in drug-resistant CPSP patients only. DBS is less invasive compared with epidural stimulation and can be used in pharmacoresistant CPSP patients and appears to be well tolerated in properly selected patient populations. DBS also has the added benefit over motor cortex stimulation of being reversible and nondestructive, and stimulator settings can be modified after placement. To date, studies of DBS have shown conflicting evidence. In one study, only 2 out of 11 CPSP patients treated with DBS had mild to moderate pain relief. In another study, pain relief was achieved in 70% of CPSP patients after permanent DBS placement. rTMS has also been proven effective and safe for the treatment of CPSP. There is still a paucity of studies on the efficacy of vestibular caloric stimulation in the treatment of CPSP; however, initial findings suggest that it may have some effectiveness in improving symptoms.

CONCLUSION

There are few guidelines for the treatment of CPSP. The general consensus is to start with amitriptyline as first-line therapy. Should this not help reduce symptoms, lamotrigine, as a second-line drug may be added. Some practitioners suggest that mexiletine, fluvoxamine, and gabapentin may be other second-line therapies. For short-term pain relief, lidocaine and propofol have been recommended. For those patients who are pharmacoresistant DBS and rTMS may prove effective.

KEY POINTS TO REMEMBER

- Central post-stroke pain is a diagnosis that is considered in the setting of occurrence following ischemic or hemorrhagic stroke, with either positive or negative sensory symptoms in the same distribution.
- Medical treatment usually begins with a trial of lamotrigine, and then a second-line drug may be added.
- For severe, refractory cases, repetitive transcranial magnetic stimulation (rTMS) may be offered.

Further Reading

Attal N, Gaude V, Brasseur L, Dupuy M, Gurimand F, Parker F, Bouhassira D. Intravenous lidocaine in central pain: a double-blind, placebo-controlled, psychophysical study. *Neurology* 2000;54:564-574.

Bittar RG, Kar-Purkyastha I, Owen SL, Bear RE, Green A, Wang S, Aziz TZ. Deep brain stimulation for pain relief: a meta-analysis. *J Clin Neurosci* 2005;12:515-519.

Craig AD, Chen K, Bandy D, Reiman EM. Thermosensory activation of insular cortex. *Nat Neurosci* 2000;3:184-190.

Frese A, Husstedt IW, Ringelstein EB, Evers S. Pharmacologic treatment of central post-stroke pain. *Clin J Pain* 2006;22(3):252-259.

Hannson P. Post-stroke pain case study: clinical characteristics, therapeutic options and long-term follow-up. *Eur J Neurol* 2004;11:22-30.

Iranami H, Ymazaki A. Tramadol challenges for relief of intractable central post stroke pain. *Mayo Clin Proc* 2006;81:566-569.

Kumar B, Kalita J, Kumar G, Misra U. Central post-stroke pain: a review of pathophysiology and treatment. *Pain Med* 2009;108(5):1645-1657.

Lampl C, Yazdi K, Roper C. Amitriptyline in the prophylaxis of central poststroke pain. *Stroke* 2003;33:3030-3032.

Leijon G, Boivie J. Central post-stroke pain: a controlled trial of amitriptyline and carbamazepine. *Pain* 1989;36:27-36.

McGeoch PD, Williams LE, Lee RR, Ramchandran VS. Behavioural evidence of vestibular stimulation as a treatment for central post-stroke pain. *J Neurol Neurosurg Psychiatry* 2008;79:1298-1301.

Vestergard K, Andersen G, Gottrup H, Kristensen BT, Jensen TS. Lamotrigine for central poststroke pain: a randomized controlled trial. *Neurology* 2001;56:184-190.

Vestergard K, Andersen G, Jansen TS. Treatment of central post stroke pain with selective serotonin reuptake inhibitor. *Eur J Neurol* 1996;3(S5):169.

Yamamoto T, Katayama Y, Hirayana T, Tsubokawa T. Pharmacological classification of central post-stroke pain: comparison with the results of chronic motor cortex stimulation therapy. Pain 197;72:5-12.

5 Multiple Sclerosis Related Pain

A 52-year-old female with a past medical history of multiple sclerosis presents to clinic. She was diagnosed 10 years ago with initial symptoms that included right-sided lip numbness and a depressed gag reflex that made swallowing difficult. Three years following her initial diagnosis, she began to have severe pain in her lower lumbar region that radiated to her left foot, affecting her ability to walk. Over the last two years, she has developed chronic pain, tremor, difficulty in walking and a severe constant burning, lancinating pain in her right foot.

What do you do now?

Multiple sclerosis (MS) is usually associated with a loss of sensation; however, since the late 1800s, physicians have recognized that pain is often associated with multiple sclerosis and can at times be the heralding symptom.

Pain can occur in 29–86% of MS patients and can include neuropathic pain, dysesthetic pain and trigeminal neuralgia, as well as somatic pain mostly originating from back pain and painful spasms. Around 5% of those with MS related pain describe this as their worst symptom, and 18% identified this as one of their three worst symptoms. The chronic nature of the pain can lead to poor quality of life, compromising their ability to work; poor interpersonal relationships; and mood disorders. Although pain in MS is highly prevalent, studies have shown that the actual use of pain medications to treat symptoms falls far below the symptom frequency, and even fewer patients are sent to see pain management specialists.

Population based studies have shown that the location of pain can be quite diverse and can be either acute or chronic. The painful disorders may be due to the inflammatory lesions of MS as well as secondary to MS-related disability (Table 5.1).

One study demonstrated a correlation between pain and age, disease duration, disease course, and expanded disability status scale (EDSS). Researchers have not found a link between disease progression and pain. However, one study found that the type of MS may play a role in the type of pain experienced. It seems that those patients with relapsing-remitting MS more frequently have pain associated with L'hermitte's sign and migraine headache. Those with primary progressive MS may have a higher incidence of dysesthetic pain, low back pain, and painful nocturnal spasms.

MANAGEMENT

To date, multiple modalities have been instituted to treat the myriad of pain syndromes seen in MS. These therapies are similar for any acute or chronic pain disorder. Medication, physical therapy, behavioral therapy, occupational therapy, interventional procedures, baclofen pump placements, and surgical interventions have been employed.

Pharmacologic Treatment

Specific drug treatments include:

- Anticonvulsants such as carbamazepine, phenytoin, gabapentin, lamotrigine
- Tricyclic antidepressants (TCAs)
- Steroids
- Local anesthetics such as bupivicaine, lidocaine, and mexiletine
- Others agents such as baclofen, amantadine, misoprostol, octreotide, acetazolamide

Anticonvulsants (See Chapter 26)

Carbamazepine   Carbamazepine is an anticonvulsant that is specifically licensed for use in treatment of trigeminal neuralgia (TN). Some interpret a favorable response from carbamazepine treatment as diagnostic for trigeminal neuralgia. It has also been reported as being effective for the treatment of glossopharyngeal neuralgia, L'hermitte's sign, and paroxysmal limb pain, and in controlling painful tonic seizures. Carbamazepine is limited by its side-effect profile, and has in some studies been linked to worsened pain in the MS population.

TABLE 5-1 **Examples of Acute and Chronic Pain Syndromes**

Acute Pain Syndromes
- Trigeminal neuralgia–if present bilaterally this is pathognomonic of MS
- L'hermitte's sign
- Acute radicular pain
- Tic-like extremity pain
- Dysesthetic limb pain (continuous burning, aching or throbbing pain particularly in the legs and feet)
- Painful tonic seizures
- Optic neuritis
- Painful bladder spasms
- Headaches

Acute Pain Syndromes
- Dysesthetic extremity pain
- Painful spasticity
- Visceral pain

Phenytoin   Phenytoin is also an anticonvulsant that is licensed for use as second-line treatment of TN, if the patient has failed carbamazepine solo therapy or is intolerant to the side effects of carbamazepine. It has also been found to be effective in the treatment of paroxysmal limb pain and for controlling painful tonic seizures.

Gabapentin   Gabapentin is an anticonvulsant that is often used for the treatment of neuropathic pain disorders. It has been shown to be helpful in treating TN when added to either carbamazepine or lamotrigine therapy. Most commonly, however, gabapentin is used for treating dysesthetic pain and for relieving refractory pain. An open label study found that it was effective for treating painful spasms and reducing associated pain.

Lamotrigine   Lamotrigine is an anticonvulsant that is also used for the treatment of TN, paroxysmal limb pain, and burning pains, as well as showing some benefit in the treatment of dysesthetic limb pain.

Tricyclic Antidepressants (See Chapter 25)

Tricyclic antidepressants are not only used for the treatment of mood disorders, but are also quite beneficial in the treatment of neuropathic pain disorders, especially amitriptyline. TCAs have been used effectively for the treatment of paroxysmal limb pain.

Steroids

Steroids are commonly used as first-line therapy for exacerbations of MS. Pain associated with optic neuritis is often best relieved by steroid therapy. It has been shown that patients treated with IV methylprednisolone had more rapid recovery of visual function initially, but not maintained at 6 months; however, the difference between oral and IV steroids on the treatment of pain has not been reported.

Local Anesthetics

Lidocaine   The complete relief of pain from L'hermitte's sign, paroxysmal limb pain, and painful spasms has been noted with the use of lidocaine.

Mexiletine   Partial relief of L'hermitte's sign pain was noted in a minority of patients. However, patients with paroxysmal limb pain, thalamic pain, and pain related to spasms reported almost complete relief.

Others

Oral and Intrathecal Baclofen   The use of oral and intrathecal baclofen for the treatment of painful spasticity has been well established. It has also been effective for the treatment of trigeminal neuralgia and dysesthetic pain. Intrathecal baclofen has a reduced side-effect profile, as compared to its oral counterpart; however, oral medication therapy should be attempted first.

Amantadine   Amantadine has commonly been used for the treatment of symptoms caused by the Influenza A virus. However, due to its dopaminergic effects, it is also been used for the treatment of Parkinson's disease, fatigue caused by MS, and chronic undefined pain. There are very few studies to show its efficacy.

Misoprostol   Misoprostol is most often used to help with the healing of duodenal ulcers and gastric ulcers. Some authors have found success in treating refractory TN with a combination of carbamazepine and misoprostol, particularly in the MS population.

Octreotide   Octreotide is a somatostatin analog that is commonly used for the relief of symptoms associated with gastroenteropancreatic endocrine tumors and acromegaly. Only one case report has demonstrated MS pain relief for dysesthetic pain with use of intrathecal octreotide at a dosage of 20mcg/hr.

Acetazolamide   Acetazolamide is a carbonic anhydrase inhibitor, and most commonly used for the treatment of glaucoma, edema, epilepsy, and certain headache syndromes. It has been effective for reducing pain secondary to spasms, as well reducing the actual spasms.

Procedural and Surgical Treatment

Depending on the location of the pain, multiple interventional techniques have been used including epidural steroid injections, selective nerve root blocks, trigger point injections and joint injections. Placement of intrathecal baclofen pumps has revolutionized the treatment of spasms and pain in the MS population. For the treatment of TN, microvascular techniques and neurolysis have been utilized. Other surgical techniques employed for the treatment of pain include placement of spinal cord stimulators and thalamotomy.

- Pain can occur in 29-86% of MS patients an can include neuropathic pain, dysesthetic pain, and trigeminal neuralgia, as well as somatic pain mostly originating from back pain and painful spasms.

- Medication, physical therapy, behavioral therapy, occupational therapy, interventional procedures, baclofen pump placements, and surgical interventions have been employed.

- Multiple interventional techniques have been used, including axial epidural steroid injections, selective nerve root blocks, trigger point injections, and joint injections.

Further Reading

Beard S, Hunn A, Wright J. Treatments for spasticity and pain in multiple sclerosis: a systematic review. *Health Technol Assess* 2003;7(40): iii, ix-x, 1-111.

Boneschi FM, Colombo B, Annovazzi P, Martinelli V, et al. Lifetime and actual prevalence of pain and headache in multiple sclerosis. *Mult Scler* 2008;14:514-521.

Solaro C, Brichetto G, Amato MP, et al. The prevalence of pain in multiple sclerosis: a multi-center cross-sectional study. *Neurology* 2004;63:919.

6 Radiculopathy

A 41-year-old man is seen with a chief complaint of pain in his low back radiating into his right buttock, his right posterior thigh, the lateral aspect of his knee, the anterolateral aspect of his lower leg and into the top of his foot. He was in his usual state of health until approximately two weeks ago when, while shoveling snow, he felt a gradual onset of low back pain. He went inside and took ibuprofen and within a few hours started feeling the pain radiating down his leg, which over the course of the next two days worsened and has persisted. He has noticed some weakness with ankle dorsiflexion. He has been unable to work in his occupation as a pharmacist since this injury.

He has been sleeping poorly and is using 800 mg of ibuprofen every 4 hours around the clock. He describes his mood as frustrated and anxious. He has no loss of control of bladder or bowel and he has no "red flags." An MRI shows a large herniated disc at the L5, S1 level on the right clearly compressing the left L5 nerve root. On physical examination, he does have weakness of the extensor hallicus longus and he has a "woody" sensation to fine touch in an L5 distribution on the left. Patellar and ankle deep tendon reflexes are symmetrical. He has no saddle signs or symptoms.

What do you do now?

EPIDEMIOLOGY

The incidence of frequent or persistent low back pain in the United States has been reported to be as high as 15% of the population. Estimates are that as many as 8% of the working population in the United States may be disabled in any given year. The 1-year prevalence of back pain in the United States may be as high as 50%. Low back pain often begins early in life with symptoms typically occurring in the 35 to 55 age range. Sciatica or radicular pain may affect 2% of the population with low back pain and is seen more frequently in men than in women. Surgery for disc herniation is performed more commonly in men than in women, and worker's compensation claims in this population are more common in men than in women.

SIGNS AND SYMPTOMS

Body weight is a weak risk indicator, and radicular pain appears more commonly in taller individuals than shorter individuals. Heavy physical work, static work postures, vibration, bending, twisting, and lifting may be risk factors for low back and radicular pain. Psychological factors such as depression and anxiety as well as job dissatisfaction increase the risk of low back and radicular pain. While most episodes of low back and radicular pain are musculoskeletal or are secondary to a herniated disc or spinal stenosis, factors such as fever, weight loss, worse pain at night, history of cancer, or older age may be "red flags" which may indicate infection, cancer, or fracture and should precipitate immediate further investigation.

Neurological findings, such as weakness on physical examination might accelerate the workup process, and progressive neurological loss could be considered a medical or surgical emergency (Table 6.1).

MANAGEMENT

The natural history of low back and radicular pain is such that it usually resolves with conservative therapy over the course of weeks to months. Conservative therapy includes the use of nonopioid analgesics, physical therapy, behavioral therapy or counseling, and strict avoidance of allowing your patient to become sedentary and deconditioned. Most experts would

TABLE 6.1 **Lumbar Nerve Syndromes**

Root	Deep Tendon Reflex	Motor Weakness	Dermatome
L1	None	None	Hip, groin
L2	None	Psoas, hip adductors	Anterior thigh
L3	Patellar	Psoas, quadriceps	Buttock, anterior thigh, knee
L4	None	Tibialis anterior	Lateral thigh, anterior lower leg, dorsum of foot
L5	Ankle	Extensor hallicus longus	As L4 plus inner half of sole and medial toes

argue against having obtained an MRI even in the patient mentioned above despite his L5 weakness because, given his age, lack of red flags, and clinical presentation, and given the natural history of lumbar radiculopathy obtaining, this study does not contribute to helping to make a diagnosis or treatment. Others would argue that on the basis of his severe incapacitation by pain and his neurological findings it may be important to clearly define a diagnosis anatomically to select treatment options.

Two possible controversies in recommended treatment for the patient mentioned include selection of opioids and the use of epidural steroid injections to help manage his pain. Patients with a predominance of leg pain and who are severely symptomatic from a herniated disc can respond very well to an epidural steroid injection. The morbidity of the procedure is exceptionally low and it can help relieve symptoms, enabling physical therapy and exercise and possibly return to work in the short term. Treatment with opioids in a low risk patient may also be useful for the same reasons that the epidural steroid injections might be. Short-term use of a short acting opioid such as oxycodone with acetaminophen may be useful, in conjunction with physical therapy, behavioral medicine approaches, nonsteroidal anti-inflammatory drugs, and injection therapy. If this patient were two months out from his injury rather than two weeks then an epidural steroid injection would clearly be an option.

The final option is surgical management. It has been shown that there is little or no difference in outcome when surgical treatment is compared to conservative treatment 2 years after the injury, but surgical treatment can improve quality of life in that 2-year interval. While 2 weeks may be too early to consider a surgical option given the natural history and other options for treatment, at 2 months given strong anatomical correlation between symptoms and radiographic findings surgery may be a reasonable option.

This patient had clear concordance between his symptoms, physical exam findings, and his MRI. He responded poorly to physical therapy, NSAIDs, and other modalities such as heat and transcutaneous electrical nerve stimulation. He continued to have disabling pain despite using three 5 mg oxycodone/acetaminophen tablets per day. He got 1 month of excellent relief from an epidural steroid injection and another month of relief when this procedure was repeated, but continued to have severe radicular disabling pain. He ultimately underwent an L5, S1 laminectomy and discectomy and had complete relief of pain when he awoke in the recovery room.

KEY POINTS TO REMEMBER

- Most episodes of radiculopathy, even with MRI abnormalities, will respond to conservative management.
- For more refractory or debilitating symptoms, low dose opioids (in low risk patients) and epidural steroid injections are indicated for temporary relief while waiting for symptoms to resolve by natural history.
- When symptoms, signs, and imaging reveal concordant findings and the patient has either not responded to conservative therapy or cannot tolerate symptoms, surgery is indicated.

Further Reading

Chou R, Loeser JD, Owens DK, et al. Interventional therapies, surgery, and interdisciplinary rehabilitation for low back pain: an evidence-based clinical practice guideline from the American Pain Society. *Spine* 2009;34(10):1066-1077.

Chou R, Atlas SJ, Stanos S, Rosenquist RW. Nonsurgical interventional therapies for low back pain: a review of the evidence for an American Pain Society Clinical Practice Guideline. *Spine* 2009;34(10):1078-1093.

Weinstein JN, Lurie JD, Tosteson TD, et al. Surgical versus nonoperative treatment for lumbar disc herniation: four-year results for the Spine Patient Outcomes Research Trial (SPORT). *Spine* 1008:33(25):789-2800.

7   Brachial Plexus Injury

A 35-year-old, right-handed female with a history of a bilateral tumor in the neck presents with paraesthesias and burning pain located in the right middle, ring, and little fingers, often during the night and worsened with cold temperature.

She also complains of fatigue and pain while writing and working on a computer, and difficulty carrying things, particularly when her arm is pulled in the axial direction or when she reaches to put dishes in her cabinets. She has impaired internal rotation/adduction/extension on the right side.

Physical examination shows palpable cervical ribs bilaterally, whereby percussion in the area elicits symptoms of pain and decrease sensation in the three ulnar fingers. The strength of the first dorsal interosseous muscle and the other ulnar nerve innervated muscles is equal to the contralateral side, but she has a positive Froment's sign. Two-point discrimination is 2-3 mm in all fingers. A normal pulse in the radial artery is noted even with the arm lifted.

Electrophysiological investigation shows no abnormalities except a slightly increased F-wave. Radiographs and CT of the cervical spine show bilateral cervical ribs articulating against a bone prominence on the cranial surface of the first rib. The cervical rib with the "pseudoarthrotic" bony formation slightly dislocates the lower part of the brachial plexus ventrally.

What do you do now?

The patient in this case presents with a brachial plexus injury. Brachial plexus injuries can vary from being acute to chronic, with symptoms ranging from transient nerve dysfunction to complete upper extremity weakness. With more significant injuries, patients may be more likely to experience psychological distress and physical disability. Because of the many anatomical variants of the brachial plexus, these injuries may be challenging to diagnose.

EPIDEMIOLOGY

Brachial plexus injuries affect men more often than women. They are most commonly due to trauma, particularly motor cycle accidents (MCA). However, other causes can include penetrating or sports related injuries, falls, work related accidents, radiation therapy, and iatrogenic causes (i.e., first rib resection, shoulder surgery, interventional radiology).

The most common mechanism of injury is a traction injury due to forceful separation of the neck from the shoulder.

Commonly associated injuries can include dislocated shoulders, fractures of the proximal humerus, clavicle, scapula, and cervical spine, and vascular injuries to the arm. Management of these injuries may complicate the picture when diagnosing brachial plexus injury, but can also guide in determining the mechanism of injury.

DIAGNOSTIC CRITERIA

When performing the history and physical examination of a patient with a suspected brachial plexus injury, it is helpful to classify the lesion. There are many classification systems for brachial plexus lesions; however, a commonly used one is Leffert's classification system (Table 7.1), which is based on the etiology and level of the injury. It is important to remember that there is a lot of variability of the brachial plexus between people and even within the same person between sides of the body. It is also true that there may be more than one level of the brachial plexus affected by a lesion. Anatomy of the brachial plexus is detailed in Table 7.2.

Pain is a common symptom of brachial plexus injuries, in particular, those affecting the preganglionic fibers. Diagnostic clues for preganglionic lesions

TABLE 7.1 **Leffert Classification of Brachial Plexus Injuries**

Classification	Etiology	Level of the Injury
I	Open (usually from stabbing)	
II	Closed (usually from MCA)	
IIa		Supraclavicular Preganglionic–nerve root avulsion Postganglionic–traction injuries
IIb		Infraclavicular
IIc		Combined
III	Radiotherapy induced	
IV	Obstetric	
IVa		Upper root (Erb's Palsy)
IVb		Lower root (Klumpke's Palsy)
IVc		Mixed

Source: Leffert RD, Brachial plexus injuries. *New Engl J Med* 1974;291:1059-1067.

include signs and symptoms of injury affecting the rhomboids or serratus anterior. Fasciculations may be seen in the paraspinal muscles if the lesions have become chronic. Patients with T1 root involvement may suffer from ipsilateral Horner's syndrome (ptosis, miosis, and anhidrosis on the affected side), as the lesion at this levels often involves the T1 sympathetic ganglion.

Symptoms often include the following:

- Severe constant pain that is often described as crushing, with episodically severe attacks shooting down the arm.
- Bizarre sensations, hyperalgesia, dysesthesia, and allodynia can occur. Studies have shown that many of the symptoms of sensory hypersensitivity, referred sensations, and motor disturbances following deafferentation may not only occur because of synaptic reorganization at the level of the subcortical and cortical structures, but may also be due to reorganization at the spinal cord level.
- Myoclonic jerks in the affected extremity.
- Paralysis and numbness in the affected extremity.

Investigative Testing

Radiographic Images

X-ray images of the clavicle and cervical spine may help to elucidate any bone abnormalities that may be causing the lesion. However, visualization of the soft tissue structures including the brachial plexus is difficult, and this cannot be determined using this imaging technique.

Magnetic resonance imaging is the most sensitive imaging technique to detect brachial plexus injury as it allows for visualization of the causative pathology. Such pathology may include infiltrating tumors, compressive

TABLE 7.2 **Anatomy of the Brachial Plexus**

Level of the Plexus	Root	Nerve	Structure Innervated
Root	C3,4,5	Phrenic	Ipsilataral hemidiaphragm
Root	C5	Dorsal scapular	Rhomboids
Root	C5,6,7	Long thoracic	Serratus anterior
Upper trunk	C5,6	Subclavius	Subclavius
Upper trunk	C5,6	Suprascapular	Supraspinatus, infraspinatus
Lateral cord	C5,6	Lateral pectoral	Clavicular and sternocostal heads pectoralis major and minor
Medial cord	C6,7,8	Medial pectoral	Sternocotal head pectoralis major, pectoralis minor
Medial cord		Medial brachial cutaneous	Medial arm above the elbow
Medial cord		Medial antebrachial cutaneous	Medial forearm
Posterior cord	C5,6,7	Upper subscapular	Subscapularis
Posterior cord	C6,7,8	Thoracodorsal	Latissimus dorsi
Posterior Cord	C5,6,7	Lower subscapular	Subscapularis, teres major

Source: Gregory J, Cowey A, Jones M, Pickard S, Ford D. The anatomy, investigations and management of adult brachial plexus injuries. *Orthopaedics and Trauma* 2009;23(6):420-432.

tumors, radiation injury, idiopathic brachial neuritis, and vasculitic granulomatous disorders. T2 weighted images are able to detect edema in and/or around the brachial plexus correlating with injury.

Histamine Test

Rarely used today, this test is helpful for differentiating preganglionic versus postganglionic injury. A drop of histamine is placed on the skin and the skin is scratched through the histamine. With an intact nerve, vasodilation, wheal formation, and a flare response (mottled reddening around the area of skin injury) will occur. With nerve damage proximal to the dorsal root ganglion, the normal response will occur in an area of skin that has anesthesia. If the lesion is distal to the dorsal root ganglion, there will be vasodilation and wheal formation in the anesthetized skin, but no flare response, because this is an axon mediated response that requires an intact functioning axon along the entire course of the nerve to the cell body.

Electrophysiology

Electromyography (EMG) and nerve conduction studies (NCS) are very useful for confirming the diagnosis, localizing the lesion, and quantifying the degree of axonal loss that may be occurring. An initial study should be performed at 3–4 weeks after the initial injury, as denervation changes can occur as early as 10–14 days after the trauma, but can take up to 40 days before they are seen on studies. Motor responses are affected before sensory responses; thus, early signs of damage may be seen as a reduction in the amplitude of the compound muscle action potential. The sensory nerve action potential (SNAP) can indicate if a lesion is pre- or postganglionic. If the SNAP is absent or reduced, then the lesion is distal to the dorsal root ganglion. On EMG, denervation signs may be seen as fibrillation potentials in the affected muscle.

MANAGEMENT

Pharmacologic Treatment

Persistent brachial plexus pain is often treated in a fashion similar to neuropathic pain. Significant pain is more common with total plexus injuries, especially, as stated above, with root avulsions. Pain lasting greater than 6 months indicates a greater risk of poor prognosis regarding neurologic recovery. Controlling pain can help to improve the mood of the patient and facilitate rehabilitation. Only one third of patients tend to report significant relief of pain with medications. Treatment with a combination of nonsteroidal anti-inflammatory drugs, tricyclic antidepressants, anticonvulsants, and oral or transdermal opioids is the often the mainstay of therapy.

Nonpharmacologic Treatment

Physiotherapy is an important aspect of treating not only the pain associated with these injuries, but also the functional capacity of the patient. The goal of therapy should be to maintain passive motion and to strengthen the affected muscles.

Chronic edema may develop due to dependent edema, loss of sympathetic tone to the vasculature, and soft tissue injury. Elevation of the limb, bracing, and compression garments can be used to reduce the edema and help to relieve stiffness and pain in the limb. Counseling, biofeedback, hypnosis, acupuncture, and transcutaneous nerve stimulation have all been used with varying degrees of effectiveness.

Procedural and Surgical Treatment

Severe cases of pain may require interventional therapy. A continuous brachial plexus block is one procedure that can be considered to achieve pain relief for prolonged periods of time. Transcutaneous nerve stimulation may also be tried.

For some time now, severe cases of brachial plexus injury pain have been treated with dorsal root entry zone (DREZ) ablation or the use of implantable dorsal root stimulators. On average, studies on the effectiveness of DREZ ablation have shown that 77% of patients have greater than 75% pain reduction, 68% have 25–75% pain reduction, and 11% have less than 25% pain reduction. This effect appears to be long lasting, up to at least 63 months, as was seen in one follow up study.

Multiple surgical modalities are used to help improve both pain and functionality. Early surgical therapy may help to reduce the morbidity due to pain and decreased function. Among these techniques are neurolysis, nerve grafting, and nerve transfer. The results of these procedures have markedly advanced with the use of newer microsurgical techniques. Explanation of each procedure is beyond the scope of this chapter; however, careful and early consideration of these procedures may prove beneficial.

KEY POINTS TO REMEMBER

- Brachial plexus injuries are most commonly due to trauma, of which motorcycle accidents are the most common.
- The most common mechanism of injury is a traction injury due to forceful separation of the neck from the shoulder.
- Significant pain is more common with total plexus injuries, especially, as stated above, with root avulsions. Pain lasting greater than 6 months indicates a greater risk of poor prognosis regarding neurologic recovery.
- Treatment with a combination of nonsteroidal anti-inflammatory drugs, tricyclic antidepressants, anticonvulsants, and oral or transdermal opioids is the often the mainstay of therapy.
- Physiotherapy is an important aspect of treating not only the pain associated with these injuries, but also the functional capacity of the patient.
- Severe cases of brachial plexus injury pain have been treated with dorsal root entry zone (DREZ) ablation or the use of implantable dorsal root stimulators.

Further Reading

Bertelli JA, Ghizoni MF. Pain after avulsion injuries and complete palsy of the brachial plexus: the possible role of nonavulsed roots in pain generation. *Neurosurgery* 2008;62(5):1104-1114.

Finnerup NB, Norrbrink C, Fuglsang-Frederiksen A, et al. Pain, referred sensations, and involuntary muscle movements in brachial plexus injury. *Acta Neurol Scand* 2010;121:320-327.

Gregory J, Cowey A, Jones M, Pickard S, Ford D. The anatomy, investigations and management of adult brachial plexus injuries. *Orthopaedics and Trauma* 2009;23(6):420-432.

Leffert RD. Brachial plexus injuries. *New Engl J Med* 1974; 291:1059-1067.

Leffert RD. Brachial plexus injuries in the adult. In: Norris TR, ed. Orthopaedic knowledge update: shoulder and elbow 2. *J Am Acad Orthop Surg* 2002:394.

Vranken J, van der Vegt MH; Zuurmond W, Pijl AJ, Dzoljic M. Continuous brachial plexus block at the cervical level using a posterior approach in the management of neuropathic cancer pain. *Reg Anesth Pain Med* 2001;26:572-575.

8 Superficial Radial Nerve Injury

A 25-year-old man presents to your office with pain over the dorsal and radial surfaces of the distal wrist and hand. He was well until two weeks ago when he presented at a university hospital with acute appendicitis and had his IV line started in this region by a medical student. He remembers having horrible, severe pain at the time of the IV insertion, and that his IV was removed immediately following his surgery because his pain was so severe. The IV was transferred to a different site; however, the pain at the insertion site has not abated. On physical examination, he has a numb area surrounding the anatomical snuffbox. Motor and sensory examinations of the upper extremity are otherwise normal.

What do you do now?

This young man has an injury of the superficial radial nerve or a branch of the superficial radial nerve, which innervates the radial half of the dorsum and two-and-a-half digits of the wrist and hand. This nerve is in close proximity to the cephalic vein, which winds upward from the dorsal venous network around the border of the wrist and forearm, and receives tributaries from both the dorsal and ventral surfaces of the hand, and thus there is often a large bifurcation directly above the superficial radial nerve. This bifurcation has frequently been called the "intern's vein" because it is often a very large vessel which can be alluring to novice venipuncturists. The nerve itself is very superficial and can be located directly subcutaneously, and most people have experienced the sensation of banging the distal end of the dorsolateral radius and having neuropathic pain from trauma to this superficial radial nerve. The superficial radial nerve has no motor innervation.

MANAGEMENT

Injury to the superficial radial nerve is not an uncommon sequela to venipuncture over the cephalic vein. It can result in severe pain, which is usually temporary, but can result in a chronic pain syndrome. It is a purely neuropathic pain syndrome and can usually be managed with optimal doses of gabapentin up to 3600 mg per day in divided doses, or pregabalin up to 450 mg per day in divided doses. It may be necessary to include an antidepressant such as duloxetine up to 60 mg per day. This pain may respond to nonsteroidal anti-inflammatory drugs, and is also likely to respond to opioids in certain severe cases. Injection of steroids over the nerve in the most painful site, along with a local anesthetic, may help resolve the symptoms, and if allodynia is present, which it often is, these symptoms may be amenable to treatment with lidocaine patches or other topical analgesics. The prognosis for a complete recovery is good, but if this pain is still present unabated 2 years after injury, it is unlikely that it will resolve.

KEY POINTS TO REMEMBER

- The superficial radial nerve lies very close to the skin surface and underlies the large bifurcation of the cephalic vein in the dorsolateral aspect of the hand and wrist.
- This nerve can be easily injured during venipuncture, and this bifurcation is especially alluring to novice venipuncturists.
- The pain is usually self-limiting following injury to this nerve but can occasionally be long lasting.
- The pain from superficial radial nerve neuralgia is usually manageable with the usual antineuropathic pain analgesics.

Further Reading

Narouze, SN, ed. *Atlas of Ultrasound-Guided Procedures in Interventional Pain Management* Springer, New York, 2011. See Part 6, 337–343.
DOI: 10.1007/978-1-4419-1681-5_26

Braidwood AS. Superficial radial neuropathy. *J Bone and Joint Surg Br* 1975;57-B(3):380.

Terzis JK, Konofaos P. Radial nerve injuries and outcomes: our experience. *Plast Reconstr Surg* 2011;127(2):739–751.

9 Post-Thoracotomy Pain (Acute and Chronic Pain)

A 65-year-old female presented to the pain clinic with complaints of severe pain in and around a thoracotomy scar. She rated her pain as 12/10 on a visual analog scale (VAS), describing it as burning in character and associated with shooting, tingling, and electric-like sensations. Exacerbating factors were prolonged sitting, standing, or walking. The patient stated that she had great discomfort with wearing her bra and tight-fitting clothing. She states that she had undergone right lower lobectomy for adenocarcinoma of the lung 10 months prior to presentation. On physical examination, the scar was well healed and measured 5 cm in length on the left inferolateral chest wall.

What do you do now?

Persistent post-thoracotomy pain syndrome (PTPS) is one of the most prevalent sources of chronic postoperative pain. Up to 20–70% of patients may complain of symptoms consistent with post-thoracotomy pain. Not only does the pain lead to feelings of intolerable discomfort and changes in mood, but in the postoperative period can cause significant decreases in respiration secondary to splinting, leading to poor sputum clearance and reduced ventilatory capacity. Adequate analgesia perioperatively has been shown to significantly decrease these complications both in the perioperative period as well as more long term. Studies have shown that when proper analgesia is used, chronic pain does not usually last longer than 2 months and recurring pain after resolution of the postoperative pain was most likely (95%) due to recurrence of tumor. They also showed that there was a small group that continued to have decreasing pain over an 8-month period of time that was not due to tumor recurrence.

The International Association for the Study of Pain (IASP) definition of chronic pain after thoracotomy is "Pain that recurs or persists along a thoracotomy scar at least 2 months following surgical procedure." The time period that this definition uses has been contentious and some will use 1 month, 2 months, 6 months, or even later. Risk factors for chronic post-thoracotomy pain include: younger age, female gender, increased or uncontrolled perioperative pain, care and timing of analgesia, history of radiation or chemotherapy, history of chronic pain prior to surgery, tumor recurrence, and psychosocial factors.

Treatments and prevention of post-thoracotomy pain have been targeted at three different times: preoperative, intraoperative, and postoperative. Those factors in the preoperative period include the age and gender of the patient, history of chronic pain, and genetic susceptibility to developing chronic pain. The one factor that may be treated in the preoperative category is to develop an effective pain management strategy for chronic pain.

Intraoperative factors leading to post-thoracotomy pain include: location of surgery, incision type, whether video-assisted thoracic surgery (VATS) was used, use of interpleural or paravertebral block and intercostal block, use of thoracic epidural anesthesia, cryoanalgesia, and preemptive analgesia.

Few studies have been performed, specifically prospective studies, to indicate which surgical type and incision type will decrease the incidence of chronic pain following thoracotomy. What can be said from the studies that have been performed is that if there is intraoperative visualization of nerve damage, then risk is increased. This appears to be also true regarding any confirmation of whether VATS utilization decreases the incidence of PTPS.

Intraoperative analgesia, has again, been understudied in this population. Some cursory studies have found that the timing of intercostal nerve blocks has not changed risk of PTPS. However, randomized double-blind studies have been performed for use of thoracic epidural anesthesia intraoperatively by comparing epidural only versus epidural with IV ketamine and showed that risk PTPS did not decrease. As intraoperative findings were not indicating any significant change in risk for developing PTPS, preemptive analgesia was targeted as a possible prevention. Again, there is a paucity of studies and there is no conclusive evidence that preemptive analgesia decreases risk.

DIAGNOSTIC CRITERIA

Diagnosis is done by careful history and physical exam with a history of recent or inciting event including thoracotomy. MRI or CT scan of the chest must be done to rule out recurrence of tumor.

MANAGEMENT

In spite of the conflicting evidence on whether the aforementioned techniques decrease risk of PTPS, the current standard of care is to use multimodal anesthesia employing systemic nonopioids and local anesthetics. Intraoperatively, thoracic epidural anesthesia and continuous paravertebral blocks are the regional techniques used. Treating those who, in spite of these efforts, continue on to chronic post-thoracotomy includes the use of topical anesthetics for allodynia, anticonvulsants, antidepressants, and opioid therapy. For those with retractable disease, injection therapy with local anesthetic and steroid therapy using a selective nerve root block may prove to be beneficial as may thoracic epidural steroid injections. For severe pain, spinal cord stimulation may be trialed.

KEY POINTS TO REMEMBER

- Persistent post-thoracotomy pain syndrome (PTPS) is one of the most prevalent sources of chronic postoperative pain. Up to 20-70% of patients may complain of symptoms consistent with post-thoracotomy pain.
- MRI or CT scan of the chest must be done to rule out recurrence of tumor.
- The current standard of care is to use multimodal anesthesia employing systemic nonopioids and local anesthetics.
- Intraoperatively, thoracic epidural anesthesia and continuous paravetebral blocks are the regional techniques used.
- For those with retractable disease, injection therapy with local anesthetic and steroid therapy using a selective nerve root block may prove to be beneficial as well as thoracic epidural steroid injections. For severe pain, spinal cord stimulation may be trialed.

Further Reading

Kanner R, Martini N, Foley KM. Nature and incidence of post-thoracotomy pain. *Proceedings of the American Academy of Oncology* 1982;1:Abstract 590.

Keller SM, Carp NZ, et al. Chronic post-thoracotomy pain. *J Cardiovasc Surg (Torino)* 1994;35(6 Suppl 1):161-164.

Suzuki M, Haraguti S, Sugimoto K, Kikutani T, Shimada Y, Sakamoto A. Low-dose intravenous ketamine potentiates epidural analgesia after thoracotomy. *Anesthesiology* 2006;105(1):111-119.

Wenk M, Schug S. Perioperative pain management after thoracotomy. *Curr Opin Anaesthesiol* 2011;(24):8-12.

Wildgaard K, Ravn J, Kehlet H. Chronic post-thoracotomy pain: a critical review of pathogenic mechanisms and strategies for prevention. *Eur J Cardiothorac Surg* 2009;36:170-180.

10 Dental Pain

A 38-year-old woman presents in your office with severe pain in her right jaw. Her pain began approximately 2 months ago when she was receiving a local anesthetic injection at her dentist for a new crown. She noted that she had severe pain when the needle was positioned, which worsened with injection. Her pain resolved during the procedure but returned within a few hours and has been severe and refractory to treatment with ibuprofen and oxycodone-acetaminophen combinations. She has been back to her dentist a number of times and had a second opinion from another dentist, neither of whom could tell her what happened or how to treat it. Her original dentist has advised her to see a psychiatrist because she is so anxious. She has severe pain and is wondering what is going on and what to do.

What do you do now?

This patient is suffering from dental pain. Her painful region is located in the lower jaw and involves the cuspid, the first bicuspid, the second bicuspid, and first molar and is innervated by the inferior alveolar nerve.

SIGNS AND SYMPTOMS

The inferior alveolar nerve is commonly anesthetized in dental practice for anesthesia of the mandibular teeth. The inferior alveolar nerve is one of the three branches of the mandibular nerve which is itself a branch (V3) of the trigeminal nerve (cranial nerve V). The nerve enters the mandibular foramen in the proximal mandible, passes through the mandibular canal, and appears on the chin as the mental nerve.

Branches of the mandibular nerve divide into sensory and motor fibers. Motor fibers supply the four muscles of mastication; the temporalis, masseter, and medial and lateral pterygoids, but not the buccinator, which is supplied by the facial nerve. The three sensory branches of the mandibular nerve to the face are the auriculotemporal, the inferior alveolar, and the buccal nerves. Once the inferior alveolar nerve exits the mandible through the mental foramen its name changes to the mental nerve, which innervates the skin of the chin and the lower lip. Within the mandible, it supplies the mandibular (lower) teeth with sensory branches that form the inferior dental plexus and give off small branches that innervate the gingiva and the teeth.

Injuries to the inferior alveolar nerve, as well as the nasal palatine nerve, which is a branch of the maxillary nerve or the second division of the trigeminal nerve, the maxillary nerve itself, are not uncommon during dental procedures. The inferior alveolar nerve, or other nerves that innervate the teeth, can be injured during local anesthetic injection either by direct trauma from the needle or via intraneuronal injection of local anesthetic. Severe pain occurring during injection should be terminated to prevent injury to the nerve from pressure exerted during possible intraneuronal injection. Root canal and other more invasive surgeries have the potential of placing the nerve or the dental plexus, a labyrinth of fine nerves innervating the teeth, in jeopardy of trauma and injury. As with other pure neuropathic pain syndromes, the pain from inferior alveolar neuralgia can be unrelenting and severe.

MANAGEMENT

Treatment includes antineuropathic pain medications; such as gabapentin or pregabalin at optimal dosages of 3600 mg per day or 450 mg per day respectively with the addition of an antidepressant such as duloxatine at a target dose of 60 mg per day. Opioids may be necessary to help control this pain as well. These three classes of neuropathic analgesics—antidepressants, anticonvulsants, and opioids—can be effective at least 50% of the time in controlling neuropathic pain.

There may be trigger points in the muscles of mastication that limit jaw opening and use and may be amenable to trigger point injection for both improvement in function and analgesia. These muscles may also respond to physical therapy, just like any other muscles in the body. There are talented therapists who are skilled in the management of these injuries and can be effective in ameliorating pain and improving function.

Anxiety and depression occur commonly in patients with severe untreated pain, particularly neuropathic pain, which can be unrelenting and excruciating. Referral to a mental health provider can be essential in effective management when combined with appropriate pharmacological and procedural management, but not usually as a singular vector of treatment when there is clearly a neuropathic injury. As a last resort, there are case reports of alveolar nerve electrical stimulation with a peripheral nerve stimulator being employed successfully in the management of refractory cases of inferior alveolar neuralgia.

KEY POINTS TO REMEMBER

- Injury to branches of the trigeminal nerve (particularly V2 and V3) is not an uncommon occurrence during even minor dental procedures and can result in severe neuropathic pain.
- Pharmacological treatment of neuropathic pain involves utilization of optimal doses of antidepressants, anticonvulsants, and opioids and is effective greater than 50% of the time in controlling this pain.
- Treatment should include, as always, procedural, pharmacological, and behavioral and physical medicine approaches to management.

Further Reading

Beaulieu P, Lussier D, Porreca F, Dickenson EH, eds. *Pharmacology of Pain*. IASP Press, International Association for the Study of Pain, Seattle, WA, 2010.

DuPont JS. Neuritic toothache. *Gen Dent* 2001;49(2):178-181.

Fishman CM, Ballantyne JC, Rathmell JP, eds. *Bonica's Management of Pain*, 4th ed. Lippincott Williams & Wilkins, Baltimore, MD, Philadelphia, PA, 2010.

11 Trigeminal Neuralgia and Atypical Facial Pain

A 62-year-old woman was diagnosed with trigeminal neuralgia with continued, severe, left-sided, stabbing pain in her left cheek and jaw for the past 2 years, which has been significantly worse in the last few months. She has had an initial work-up and has been diagnosed with trigeminal neuralgia. She has been treated in the past with carbamazepine, but the efficacy has diminished in the last few months. The pain is now interfering with her quality of life, such that it is difficult for her to work as a telemarketer. Her past medical history is significant for hypertension, for which she is on a beta blocker. She presents for pain control.

What do you do now?

The patient is suffering from trigeminal neuralgia (TN), which is not uncommon in the elderly, is more prevalent in women, and tends to involve the second and/or third division of the trigeminal nerve predominantly. She is currently not having substantial relief on carbamazepine, and her goal is to have decreased pain such that she is able to participate in work and have a better quality of life.

TRIGEMINAL NEURALGIA

Epidemiology

Trigeminal neuralgia is more common in patients in their 60s, affects women slightly more than men, and affects the second and third divisions of the trigeminal nerve predominantly.

Diagnostic Criteria

The diagnosis of craniofacial pain is often difficult because of its similarity to other disease processes. The International Association for the Study of Pain's definition of trigeminal neuralgia is "sudden, usually unilateral, severe, brief, stabbing, recurrent pain in the distribution of one or more branches of the fifth cranial nerve." When a patient presents with facial pain, the diagnosis should include clinical history, physical exam, and radiological evidence to exclude intracranial lesions. Precise diagnosis is essential, as it has various diagnostic and prognostic implications.

Currently, clinical cases of trigeminal neuralgia can be classified into the following categories:

- *Classical or typical trigeminal neuralgia*, which is a sudden, usually unilateral, severe, brief, stabbing, recurrent pain in the distribution of one or more branches of the fifth cranial nerve. Over 90% of TN patients fall into this category. It is often termed an idiopathic syndrome, meaning the underlying cause of the disorder is not known.
- *Atypical or nonclassical trigeminal neuralgia*, which is often described as a constant, burning, gnawing pain in the same distribution. This term is used for cases associated with multiple sclerosis and other causes such as tumors or vascular anomalies, which can be identified on cranial imaging.

TABLE 11.1 Secondary Causes of Trigeminal Neuralgia

ophthalmologic disease
dental disease
sinus disease, diseases of the ear canal
headaches
other neuralgias
giant cell arteritis, aneurysms
neoplasia

When diagnosing trigeminal neuralgia, other causes of facial pain should be excluded (Table 11.1).

MANAGEMENT

If a secondary cause is identified, it should be treated appropriately. If a patient has a diagnosis of trigeminal neuralgia without a secondary cause, medical management should be instituted. Carbemazepine is likely to be beneficial in 70% of patients and remains the gold standard. The incidence of side effect is often higher in the elderly and may limit its usefulness in this population at times. Hematologic adverse reactions include lowering of the white cell count and megaloblastic anemia associated with folic acid deficiency. Some patients may develop an allergic rash. Carbemazepine has a number needed to treat (NNT) of 2.5 for 50% pain relief. If carbamazepine is ineffective, other anticonvulsant drugs are the treatment of choice. Although anticonvulsant drugs (ACDs) have been evaluated for neuropathic pain states, there are no trials comparing different ACDs specifically for trigeminal neuralgia. The current first-line treatment in regard to ACDs includes phenytoin, gabapentin, lamotrigine, topiramate, oxcarbazepine, zonisamide, and similar combination regimens (see Table 26.2).

Other pharmacological therapies include baclofen, which has been shown to be effective in altering input at the trigeminal brainstem level as well as having analgesic properties. In addition, treatment with tricyclic antidepressants including amitriptyline and nortriptyline has been shown to be effective in other neuropathic pain states (see Table 25.1). Clonazepam, a benzodiazepine with anticonvulsant properties, in several studies in the mid-1970s demonstrated it also suppressed pain attacks in trigeminal neuralgia.

The side-effect profile of various medication treatment options can limit its utility, most notably in elderly patients. The tricyclic antidepressants can lead to tachycardia or can prolong the QT interval, so electrocardiographic monitoring is essential. In addition, they can cause anticholinergic side effects including dry mouth, constipation, sedation, cognitive dysfunction, and urinary retention, which can limit their usefulness in this population.

Procedural and Surgical Treatment

If medical management fails, there are numerous procedural treatments for trigeminal neuralgia. The pathophysiology responsible for any of the signs and symptoms of trigeminal neuralgia is not new; however, there is increasing evidence that injury to the gasserion ganglion, or trigeminal nerve is an important factor. There is a strong suggestion that chronic nerve compression injury might induce changes in the nerve, resulting in the symptoms of TN and possibly vascular compression. Therefore, many of the procedural and surgical treatment options are focused on this pathology. These include lesioning the gasserian ganglion percutaneously via chemical, thermal (radiofrequency), or mechanical lesioning. The main disadvantage of ablative techniques is that is contraindicated in patients with ophthalmic division pain, they can produce numbness, there is a high recurrence rate, and there is a risk for Anesthesia Dolorosa, a severe, constant pain in the numb area of the face.

Exploration of the trigeminal root in the posterior fossa is a major operation with a risk for mortality and major morbidity. An alternative procedure is microvascular decompression, which is based on the theory of neurovascular compression. Microvascular decompression of the trigeminal nerve is offered to patients who have unrelenting pain and do not want to live with facial numbness. This procedure limits the risk for facial sensory loss, dysesthesias, and Anesthesia Dolorosa, which are frequently associated with sensory rhizotomies.

ATYPICAL FACIAL PAIN

There are other forms of neuralgia and atypical facial pain including glossopharyngeal neuralgia. These are rare conditions, and data is limited on their prevalence. Workup is similar to trigeminal neuralgia, including magnetic resonance imaging; however, their treatment in regard to medication is similar.

Further Reading

Chandra B. The use of clonazepam in the treatment of tic douloureux (a preliminary report). *Proc Aust Assoc Neurol* 1976;13:119-122.

Fromm GH, Terrence CF. Comparison of L-baclofen and racemic baclofen in trigeminal neuralgia. *Neurology* 1987;37(11):1725-1728.

Fromm GH, Terrence CF, Chattha AS. Baclofen in the treatment of trigeminal neuralgia: double-blind study and long-term follow-up. *Ann Neurol* 1984;15(3):240-244.

Merskey H, Bogduk M. *Classification of Chronic Pain*. IASP Press, Seattle, 1994.

Scrivani SJ, Mehta N, Mathews ES, Maciewicz R. Clinical criteria for trigeminal neuralgia. *Oral Surg Oral Med Oral Pathol Oral Radiol Endod*. May 2004;97(5):544; author reply 544-545.

Wiffen P, McQuay H, Carroll D, Jadad A, Moore A. Anticonvulsant drugs for acute and chronic pain. *Cochrane Database Syst Rev* 2000(2):CD001133.

Zakrzewska JM. Diagnosis and differential diagnosis of trigeminal neuralgia. *Clin J Pain* 2002;18(1):14-21.

Zakrzewska JM. Facial pain: neurological and non-neurological. *J Neurol Neurosurg Psychiatry* 2002;72(Suppl 2):ii27-ii32.

Zakrzewska JM, Chaudhry Z, Nurmikko TJ, Patton DW, Mullens EL. Lamotrigine (lamictal) in refractory trigeminal neuralgia: results from a double-blind placebo controlled crossover trial. *Pain* 1997;73(2):223-230.

Zakrzewska JM, Patsalos PN. Long-term cohort study comparing medical (oxcarbazepine) and surgical management of intractable trigeminal neuralgia. *Pain* 2002;95(3):259-266

12 Phantom Pain

A 34-year-old male with a history of a right arm amputation due to a motor vehicle accident, presents to the pain clinic with severe, constant pain localized in the phantom hand and fingers. The phantom arm is located with the hand and fingers extended in front of his chest. The pain waxes and wanes. During episodes of severe pain, he describes the pain as lancinating. He has tried multiple therapies including antidepressants, anticonvulsants, and opioids. Other than evidence of the site of limb amputation, the rest of his physical exam is within normal limits.

What do you do now?

Phantom pain is described as pain or dysesthesia that is caused by interruption or discontinuation of sensory nerve impulses by destroying or injuring the sensory nerve fibers after amputation or deafferentation. This should be differentiated from telescoping, which is the perception of feeling the distal limb more proximally, and stump pain, which is pain at the site of removal. The usual cause of pain is due to trauma or surgical manipulation. The incidence of phantom limb pain varies across studies and is on the order of 2–80%; however, the average appears to be between 40–70%.

The pain is often described as occurring in the first week after amputation, but can occur months or even years later. The earlier and more severely the symptoms occur, the poorer the prognosis for improvement. In most cases, about 5–10% of those with phantom limb pain will have severe pain. The pain is usually intermittent, lasting a few minutes and up to a few hours, localizing mostly to the distal parts of the missing extremity, and is described as shooting, pricking, and burning. Other descriptives have been used, as well, to describe the pain.

The exact mechanism for phantom pain is still unclear. There are a myriad of hypotheses, including the theory that reorganization of the cortical sensory fiber representation occurs following deafferentation or amputation. Although less well studied, to date, these changes may also be seen in the thalamus, brainstem, and/or the spinal cord. More likely is that there are a series of changes that occur first in the periphery, spreading up the spinal cord and terminating with cortical reorganization. The details of this process are beyond the scope of this chapter.

MANAGEMENT

Pharmacologic Treatment

Medical treatment is first-line therapy for patients suffering from phantom limb pain. Tricyclic antidepressants and sodium channel blockers are the most commonly used medications, and those that have proven to be the most beneficial for neuropathic pain in multiple randomized-controlled studies. One study by Bone et al. in 2002 showed that after six weeks of treatment, gabapentin was more beneficial at reducing phantom limb pain than placebo. Should more conventional therapies not provide sufficient relief, the patient should next be trialed on opiates.

Other nontraditional medical therapies include NMDA receptor antagonists, calcitonin, beta blockers, topical capsaicin, intrathecal opioids and anesthetic blocks. IV ketamine has been shown to reduce pain, hyperalgesia, and wind-up-like pain. Calcitonin has been shown to significantly reduce phantom pain when used intravenously in the early postoperative phase.

Nonpharmacologic Treatment

Early nonmedical treatments that have also been used include physical therapy, massage, manipulation, transcutaneous electrical nerve stimulation (TENS) units, acupuncture, ultrasound, and hypnosis. Using these therapies limits the risk of side effects and complications that may be seen with use of medical therapy.

Of increasing prevalence are surgical therapies to treat phantom pain. These include techniques such as dorsal root entry zone lesions (DREZ) and placement of spinal cord stimulators. Therapies previously performed that have since fallen out of favor include sympathectomy, stump revision, and cordotomy.

KEY POINTS TO REMEMBER

- Phantom limb and phantom limb pain that severely affects patients to the point of disrupting their lives, is apparent in a minority of patients.
- Mechanisms underlying phantom pain pathology include a complex interplay of changes involving peripheral nerves, spinal cord plasticity, brainstem, thalamus, and cortical reorganization.
- Medical therapy should be tried initially and should not be considered a failure until opioid therapy has been trialed.
- Surgical therapy including spinal cord stimulator placement and DREZ lesions should be reserved for refractory cases.

Further Reading

Bone M, Critchley P, Buggy DJ. Gabapentin in postamputation phantom limb pain: a randomized, double-blind, placebo-controlled, cross-over study. *Reg Anesth Pain Med* 2002;27(5):481-486.

Sindrup SH, Jensen TS. Efficacy of pharmacological treatments of neuropathic pain: an update and effect related to mechanism of drug action. *Pain* 1999;83:389-400.

Woolf CJ, Chong MS. Preemptive analgesia-treating postoperative pain by preventing the establishment of central sensitization. *Anesth Analg* 1993;77:362-379.

A 36-year-old male presents wheelchair-bound approximately 1 year following a T11 burst fracture with spinal cord injury and resultant paraplegia sustained in a snowmobile accident. He subsequently underwent a T10-L1 fusion with rod placement from T9 through L2. Since surgery, he has had pain at the inferior site of his rods. That pain seems to come and go and can vary between mild and severe. He describes it as an irritation, a clamping sensation, or a tight sensation. He also complains of a circumferential pain, worse on the right than on the left, at approximately the T12 or L1 level, which he describes as burning, pressure-like, and constant and severe all the time. He has been unable to tolerate cox-2 inhibitors. He has not tried other nonsteroidal anti-inflammatory drugs. He has not had relief from muscle relaxants, acetaminophen, hydrocodone, fentanyl, morphine, methadone, or meperidine. However, he does get relief from oxycodone and he is currently using sustained-release oxycodone 40 mg twice a day and short-acting oxycodone 10 mg one or two every four hours as needed and he is using approximately 10 per day.

He denies a history of alcoholism or any other substance abuse and he does not smoke cigarettes. He is unemployed and on disability. He admits to being depressed and to sleeping poorly, primarily because he has to awaken to take his pain medication and to self-catheterize his bladder. On physical examination, he had a preference for the prone position on the examination table because it was more comfortable for him. His rods hurt more when he lies in any other position. The inferior aspect of the rods could easily be palpated, the region was erythematous, and the patient reported that this was the location of some of his pain. He had variable sensation at the T11 and 12 dermatomes, and there was a clear band of allodynia with hyperalgesia at approximately the T12 level circumferentially. He occasionally had a deep, aching pain in both lower extremities below the level of his injury, but this was moderate in severity at its worst. He is requesting advice for the management of his pain.

What do you do now?

Pain following spinal cord injury is quite common. It has been estimated that between 65% and 85% of all people who sustain a spinal cord injury have ongoing pain, and a third of these report that the pain is often severe. There are a variety of different types of pain that can occur after spinal cord injury, the first being musculoskeletal. This pain is generally located at or near the sight of injury if it is related to the injury, but patients with spinal cord injury often have chronic pain related to overuse, especially patients in wheelchairs who may complain of pain in the arm or shoulder.

Patients with spinal cord injury may also have pain related to spasticity or muscle spasm. Iatrogenic pain related to surgery or hardware is not unusual. These patients may also complain of visceral pain, which can occur as a result of urinary tract infection, bowel obstruction, or kidney stones. The pain from intra-abdominal viscera in a patient with a thoracic or lumbar injury may present identically as it might in a patient without a spinal cord injury, but in patients with high thoracic or cervical cord injury, patients may present with poorly defined unpleasant sensations that are difficult to interpret.

Patients with spinal cord injury may suffer from at-level neuropathic pain usually within a few segments below their level of injury. This pain can present in a unilateral or bilateral radicular pattern and is often accompanied by allodynia or hyperalgesia. Patients with a spinal cord injury may also suffer from below-level neuropathic pain, which can be described as diffuse and may involve the entire body below the level of injury or more often a few levels below the level of the injury. Below-level pain may not occur until months or years after the initial injury and is often referred to as central pain, although the at-level spinal cord injury can also be referred to as central pain. Both the at-level and the below-level pain are typically unaffected by movement, although the at-level pain can at times be affected by movement.

MANAGEMENT

Treatment of musculoskeletal pain may be ameliorated by the use of non-steroidal anti-inflammatory drugs or acetaminophen, although nonsteroidal anti-inflammatory drugs should be used with caution because the incidence of gastrointestinal bleeding is greater in patients with spinal cord injury than it is in the general population. Muscle relaxants may be useful. Oral baclofen, zannflex, botox injections, or intrathecal baclofen can be utilized if spasticity is a significant cause of pain and/or disability.

If a specific musculoskeletal etiology of the pain can be ascertained, as it is with the patient presented above, then it may be possible to correct the anatomical cause of pain. The patient presented above had his rods in place for a year. They were clearly the source of his musculoskeletal pain, and a surgical consultation might be useful to determine whether or not those rods could be removed after this period of time, since it is likely that his spine is now stable, and this might help to relieve the musculoskeletal symptoms that he was complaining of.

The neuropathic pain expressed both at and below the level of injury can be treated with antidepressants, anticonvulsants, and opioids. Our patient had not been treated with antidepressants or anticonvulsants, and in addition he admitted, as many spinal cord patients do, to being depressed. This patient should be treated with, for example, an increasing dose of gabapentin or pregabalin and possibly duloxetine. He is currently using approximately 180 mg of morphine equivalents per day of oxycodone (assuming a 1-to-1 equianalgesic ratio). In patients with such dramatic objective evidence of a painful disorder and refractoriness to lower doses or usual doses of opioids, these doses can be increased and it may be possible that an increase in dosage up to approximately 300 mg of morphine equivalents per day might be useful.

If he failed to respond to those pharmacological and surgical interventions adequately, then it is easy to do a trial of spinal cord stimulation and this can be useful in both at-level and below-level neuropathic pain syndromes associated with spinal cord injury. Deep brain stimulation has not been shown to be particularly effective in this patient population, but there are multiple case reports of the usefulness of motor cortex stimulation, and referral to an experienced neurosurgeon might be appropriate. The use of intrathecal analgesics such as morphine, hydromorphone, clonidine, or bupivicaine as a last resort might help to provide relief. Unfortunately the intrathecal infusion of analgesics is a labor-intensive process, usually resulting in incomplete analgesia, and the occurrence of granulomatous catheter tip tumors may have an incidence as high as 50%, which may be especially dangerous in a population where patients may not feel the expansion of this tumor and where further central neurological loss may be particularly devastating.

CONCLUSION

Patients with injury to their spinal cord may be some of the most challenging of all pain patients to treat. Successful management may require special knowledge of pain etiology and an awareness of a broad array of potential treatment options.

As with all patients with chronic pain, and especially important in patients with what may be a newly acquired severely debilitating spinal cord injury, attention to emotional, situational, and social issues may be extremely helpful in improving quality of life.

KEY POINTS TO REMEMBER

- Pain following spinal cord injury is quite common and is often described as severe.
- Pain can be musculoskeletal, visceral, or neuropathic.
- Neuropathic pain may occur below-level or at-level in relation to the injury.
- Patients with neuropathic pain are often treated with anticonvulsants, antidepressants, and opioids.

Further Reading

Cardenes DD, Felix ER. Pain after spinal cord injury: a review of classification, treatment approaches, and treatment assessment. *PM R* 2009;1(12):1077-1090.

Siddall PJ. Management of neuropathic pain following spinal cord injury: now and in the future. *Spinal Cord* 2009;47(5):352-359.

Widerstrom-Noga EG, Finnerup NB, Siddall PJ. Biopsychosocial perspective on a mechanisms-based approach to assessment and treatment of pain following spinal cord injury. *J Rehabil Res Dev* 2009;46(1):1-12.

Yezierski RP. Spinal cord injury pain: spinal and supraspinal mechanisms. *J Rehabil Res Dev* 2009;46(1):95-107.

14 Ramsay Hunt Syndrome (Geniculate Neuralgia)

A 43-year-old female with a diagnosis of diabetes had a 1-week history of fever (38.5°C), ear pain, and vesicles in the right ear and neck for which she was hospitalized with a diagnosis of varicella zoster virus (VZV) infection. On the second day of the hospitalization, she developed weakness of the right facial muscles. On physical examination, the patient had a fever of 39°C, with crusted vesicular lesions especially on the neck and right ear. At rest, the facial muscles were symmetrical with normal tone. On examination, she had no movement in the right forehead, incomplete right eye closure, and an asymmetric smile. Other systemic examinations were normal.

The patient was diagnosed with Ramsay Hunt syndrome (RHS) and was started on a r egimen of methylprednisolone (1 × 100 mg IV) and acyclovir (3 × 250 mg IV). Acyclovir treatment was continued for 10 days, and methylprednisolone levels tapered to 5 mg/day after 6 days. At day 10, the skin lesions had almost cleared, and at day 30, facial paralysis partially recovered with complete eye closure with maximal effort.

What do you do now?

Ramsay Hunt syndrome is a rare entity that was first described in early 1907 by James Ramsay Hunt. There are three Ramsay Hunt syndromes, which vary dramatically from one another with the only similarity being that they were described by the same person. In this article, we will discuss Ramsay Hunt syndrome type 2, commonly known as herpes zoster oticus, which is accompanied by a peripheral facial palsy. Ramsay Hunt syndrome type 1 is known as dyssenergia cerebellaris progressive, and type 3 is a syndrome of carotid artery occlusion.

Ramsay Hunt syndrome is caused by reactivation of the herpes zoster virus within the head of the geniculate ganglion. It is defined as a peripheral facial neuropathy accompanied by erythematous vesicular rash of the ear (herpes zoster oticus) or mouth. It is the second most common cause of atraumatic peripheral facial nerve palsy.

SIGNS AND SYMPTOMS

Patients tend to present with paroxysmal pain deep within the ear. The pain will often radiate to the pinna of the ear and can then become more constant and nagging in quality. The onset of pain can precede the rash by hours and up to several days. The pain can sometimes be associated with lacrimation, nasal congestion, and salivation.

The rash is characterized as vesicular and tends to follow the distribution of the nervus intermedius. Common locations for the rash include: anterior two thirds of the tongue, soft palate, external auditory canal, and pinna. Although commonly seen, a rash may not be present on examination (zoster sine herpete). This form is characterized by peripheral facial paralysis without ear or mouth rash in light of a four-fold increase in varicella zoster virus antibody or detection of varicella zoster virus DNA in skin, blood mononuclear cells, or middle ear fluid. This has been found to occur in up to 2.4–19% of patients.

Facial paralysis can occur in any gender and at any age occurring in both children (16.7% of unilateral facial palsies) and adults with almost equal frequency, but rarer in those under the age of 6 years. In general, facial neuropathies are almost always unilateral but can be bilateral in up to 1–2% of patients. On examination, ipsilateral paresis or paralysis of the facial muscles will be seen, involving all muscles of facial expression to varying degrees. This is known as a peripheral nerve lesion, which is due to a lesion at the level of or caudal to the pontine nucleus, as opposed to one rostral to the pontine nucleus, which would cause paresis or paralysis of the contralateral lower facial muscles, known as a central facial nerve palsy. Weakness of the facial muscles tends to peak by 1 week after the onset and can become severe and even lead to complete paralysis in 52% of adults and 44% of children.

In the case of Ramsay Hunt syndrome, other cranial neuropathies are frequent and can involve, but are not limited to, neuropathies of cranial nerves V, VI, VIII, IX, and X. Up to 53% will suffer from hearing loss, which can remain persistent in up to 38%. Patients may complain of loss of sensation over the affected muscles of the face, tinnitus, dysarthria, dysphagia, vomiting, and vertigo. These contiguous cranial neuropathies have been said to occur due to the selective permeability of blood vessels to varicella zoster virus (VZV) and the vulnerability of the blood supply from small branches of the carotid artery, middle meningeal, and ascending pharyngeal system to cranial nerves.

DIAGNOSTIC CRITERIA

Clinical diagnosis is established with careful history taking, evaluation of the neurologic exam with careful consideration of cranial nerve function, and examination for evidence of lesions suggestive of herpes zoster infection.

Electrodiagnostic tests may be used, including electromyography (EMG) and nerve conduction velocity (NCV) testing, to determine the extent of facial nerve and muscle involvement. EMG of facial innervated muscles, the blink reflex, and the nerve excitability test may be used to assist with not only diagnosis but also prognosis. However, Wallerian degeneration of the motor nerve fibers takes 5–8 days after axonal injury, thus for prognostic purposes, NCVs will be of little value if performed before this time frame.

At this time, examinations of CSF and imaging studies have no real role in diagnosis of this syndrome, other than to rule out other causes of inflammation or injury to the facial nerve that may be causing symptoms. Investigations into testing of exudates from the geniculate ganglion by polymerase chain reaction for the varicella zoster virus are still under way, but may prove to be useful in differentiating facial paralysis due to Bell's palsy versus that due to Ramsay Hunt syndrome.

MANAGEMENT

The recommended treatment of RHS consists of oral steroids and acyclovir especially within 3 days of eruption of the vesicles. Almost 75% of patients experience a complete resolution of their symptoms and signs when treatment is started early. Researchers have found that if treatment is started between 4 and 7 days, the cure rate decreases to 30%. Acylovir is given orally up to a maximum dose of 4000 mg/d or intravenously at 3 × 250 mg/d for 7 to 10 days, while methylprednisolone is recommended at 1 mg/kg/d, which is tapered after 5 days. There was no difference in outcome noted between using the parenteral versus the oral formulations of acyclovir. Acyclovir has been found to exert its effect by preventing further proliferation or spread of VZV as well as perhaps decreasing the amount of otalgia associated with the syndrome. Steroids exert their effect through their anti-inflammatory role, which helps to decrease the edema associated with the neuritis caused by VZV. Together, the combination has been shown to prevent further nerve degeneration.

The treatment of pain associated with Ramsay Hunt syndrome has not been well studied or characterized. Thus, many tend to treat the pain similarly to that of postherpetic neuralgia. Please refer to chapter 3 on postherpetic neuralgia for a more complete description of these treatment strategies and their efficacy.

PROGNOSIS

A demyelinating lesion of the facial nerve may recover within days to weeks due to remyelination of the affected nerve segment by Schwann cells. However, more severe lesions that result in axonal damage and distal Wallerian degeneration will take longer to heal and recover function. The regeneration of the nerve may be incomplete, resulting in persistent paresis or paralysis, contracture of the facial muscles and synkinesis. Indicators of poor prognosis include lack of nerve excitability, complete paralysis, and age over 50.

Further Reading

Hato N, Kisaki H, Honda N, Gyo K, Murukami S, Yanagihara N. Ramsay Hunt syndrome in children. *Ann Neurol* 2000;48:254-256.

Murukami S, Hato N, Horiuchi J, et al. Treatment of Ramsay Hunt syndrome with acyclovir-prednisone: significance of early diagnosis and treatment. *Ann Neurol* 1997;41:353-357.

Murukami S, Hato N, Mizobuch M, et al. Rapid diagnosis of varicella zoster virus infection in acute facial palsy. *Neurology* 1998;51:1202-1205.

Sweeney CJ, Gilden DH. Ramsay Hunt syndrome. *J Neurol Neurosurg Psychiatry* 2001;71:149-154.

Ulusoy S, Ozkan G, Bektas D et al. Ramsay Hunt syndrome in renal transplantation recipient: a case report. *Transplant Proc* 42(2010):1986-1988.

15   Supraorbital Neuralgia

A 32-year-old woman began to suffer from right sided headaches after a motor vehicle accident in which her forehead hit the windshield. She describes her pain as a right-sided, piercing, burning pain located above the eye. The pain does not radiate to any other portion of the skull, but is sensitive to touch. The patient has been seen by her primary care provider and was diagnosed with supraorbital neuralgia after further evaluation. Post injury, she underwent a CT of the brain, which was read as normal. She was placed on amitriptyline with some benefit; however, she presents to her primary care provider's office with continued pain despite treatment.

What do you do now?

The patient's diagnosis is supraorbital neuralgia. It is caused by damage to the supraorbital nerve, which is located just superior to the eye. Patients who suffer from this condition may have suffered a history of trauma to the head, a previous black eye, or previous injury that resulted in a blow to the head. Supraorbital neuralgia was originally reported in the 1980s when two neurologists developed bitemporal headaches after one to two hours of swimming, which they later attributed to poor-fitting goggles, terming these types of headaches "swimmer's headaches."

SIGNS AND SYMPTOMS

Patients often describe pain located in the sensory area of the supraorbital nerve. The pain is usually located only on the affected side. It is often a continuous, piercing, burning-type pain, but can be paroxysmal. The pain does not have the sensory sensitivity (nausea, intolerance to light, noise, and movement) with autonomic manifestations (eye watering, nasal stuffiness, drooping of the eyelid) as seen in other headache conditions. Often, the affected area is abnormally sensitive to tactile sensation, causing hyperalgesia, allodynia, and hyperesthesia with a positive Tinel's sign.

DIAGNOSTIC CRITERIA

Diagnosis is based on history, physical exam, and normal imaging studies. The physical exam should include examining around the margins of the eye socket and the inner third of the upper rim of the eye socket, where the supraorbital neuralgia is often found. Neuroimaging tests should be normal, and a supraorbital nerve block should temporarily relieve patient's pain.

Other conditions that resemble supraorbital neuralgia should be excluded. The differential diagnosis can include:

- Other types of headaches including cluster migraines, short-lasting unilateral neuralgiform headache with conjunctival injection and tearing, sinusitis, trigeminal neuralgia.
- Skin cancer causing involvement of the periorbital sensory nerves in patients who have a history of skin cancer or a history of cutaneous malignancy.
- Other pain syndromes.

MANAGEMENT

As in other types of neuralgia, treatment is focused on medical management, procedural therapy, alternative medicine, and for cases refractory to conservative treatment, implantable stimulator devices or decompressive surgery. In cases where supraorbital neuralgia is caused by provoking stimulus, removing the offender can decrease patient's pain. This could include better-fitting helmets or swimming goggles in some cases.

Pharmacologic Treatment

Anticonvulsants such as gabapentin, pregabalin, topiramate, and others are also useful in patients with severe headaches. In addition, tricyclic antidepressants may be beneficial, as they have been found to be beneficial in other cases of neuralgias, although there are no randomized controlled trials that have demonstrated their benefit in supraorbital neuralgia. Antidepressants that help to modulate the pain pathways, such as duloxetine, may also be trialed. These medications may reduce the frequency and severity of the pain.

Nonpharmacologic Treatment

If conservative treatment with medications and injections does not seem to be beneficial, treatment with acupuncture or cognitive behavioral therapy may prove to be beneficial.

Procedural and Surgical Treatment

If a local anesthetic injection relieves the pain, a supraorbital nerve block with steroid could provide longer-term relief.

Recently, a peripheral nerve stimulating device applied to the supraorbital nerve has been shown in case reports to relieve supraorbital neuralgia (see Figure 15.1) (see chapter 29).

In severe cases, decompression of the supraorbital nerve has been attempted; however, it has not proven to be beneficial for all patients with supraorbital neuralgia. In some patients, the supraorbital nerve sits in a groove, "the supraorbital notch," whereas in other patients it runs through a small hole (the supraorbital foramen), which offers more protection at the brow of the forehead. It is said that those with a notch are more at risk of developing neuralgia, as there is less protection.

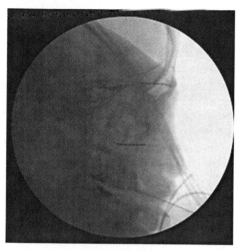

FIGURE 15.1 Supraorbital and infraorbital peripheral nerve stimulators placed in a patient with bilateral infraorbital and supraorbital neuralgia. (Courtesy of Gilbert J. Fanciullo, MD, MS, Department of Anesthesiology, Section of Pain Medicine, Dartmouth Hitchcock Medical Center, Lebanon, NH.)

CONCLUSION

Although there is lack of studies to support treatment for supraorbital neuralgia, there is evidence of treatment success for other types of neuralgia, and therefore treatment options most notably with medications are extrapolated to supraorbital neuralgia.

KEY POINTS TO REMEMBER

- Supraorbital neuralgia is an uncommon cause of facial pain.
- Pain is located in the sensory area of the supraorbital nerve and usually only on the affected side.
- Diagnosis is based on history, physical exam, and normal imaging studies.
- Medical treatment may be based on polypharmacy with anticonvulsant, tricyclic antidepressants and anticonvulsants. The side-effect profile of the medications may limit their usefulness in certain patients.
- In cases where it is caused by provoking stimulus, removing the offender can decrease patient's pain, including using better-fitting helmets or swimming goggles in some cases.

Further Reading

Adant JP, Bluth F. Endoscopic supraorbital nerve neurolysis. *Acta Chir Belg* 1999;99(4):182-184.

Amin S, Buvanendran A, Park KS, Kroin JS, Moric M. Peripheral nerve stimulator for the treatment of supraorbital neuralgia: a retrospective case series. *Cephalalgia* 2008;28(4):355-359.

Caminero AB, Pareja JA. Supraorbital neuralgia: a clinical study. *Cephalalgia* 2001;21(3):216-223.

Ducic I, Larson EE. Posttraumatic headache: surgical management of supraorbital neuralgia. *Plast Reconstr Surg* 2008;121(6):1943-1948.

O'Brien JC Jr. Swimmer's headache, or supraorbital neuralgia. *Proc (Bayl Univ Med Cent)* 2004;17(4):418-419.

Pareja JA, Caminero AB. Supraorbital neuralgia. *Curr Pain Headache Rep* 2006;10(4):302-305.

Pestronk A, Pestronk S. Goggle migraine. *N Engl J Med* 1983;308(4):226-227.

16 Glossopharyngeal Neuralgia

A 45-year-old male presents to clinic with a history of sharp pain in the back of his throat and tongue, which lasts a few minutes multiple times a day. The attacks are triggered by swallowing or drinking cold liquids, and although he has been diagnosed with glossopharyngeal neuralgia and placed on gabapentin, his symptoms persist. He presents to your clinic with pain that is affecting his quality of life, and would like further pain management.

What do you do now?

Glossopharyngeal neuralgia (GN) is a rare condition that affects the glossopharyngeal nerve (the ninth cranial nerve) and causes severe, brief, stabbing, recurrent pain in the back of the throat and tongue, the tonsils, and part of the ear (the distribution of the glossopharyngeal nerve).

EPIDEMIOLOGY

Glossopharyngeal neuralgia is a rare condition with no data on its prevalence. The mechanism may be similar to that of trigeminal neuralgia with compression of nerve roots. GN usually begins after the age of 40 and it occurs more often in men. Rarely, the cause of this disorder is a tumor in the brain or neck.

SIGNS AND SYMPTOMS

The pain is usually unilateral, but more likely to be bilateral than is trigeminal neuralgia. Its distribution is within the posterior tongue, tonsillar fossa, and pharynx, beneath the angle of the jaw, and may radiate to the inner ear or to the neck. The pain is often sharp and shooting in quality, but a dull, aching, burning pain is often present. Attacks are brief and occur intermittently, but can cause excruciating pain. The pain is often triggered by particular activities such as swallowing, contact with fluids (especially cold), yawning, talking, coughing, sneezing, and moving the head. In a minority of patients, it may also be associated with syncope and cardiac arrhythmias, as the heart rate can be affected.

DIAGNOSTIC CRITERIA

Glossopharyngeal neuralgia is distinguished from trigeminal neuralgia based on the patient's pain location, a result of clinical evaluation, physical exam, and imaging studies. If the patient has pain in the back of the throat, a local anesthetic is applied, and if the pain is eliminated, then GN is diagnosed. Prior to a final diagnosis, however, magnetic resonance imaging with gadolinium is recommended prior to rule out lesions of the brain or brainstem.

MANAGEMENT

Treatment is based on case series, as no randomized control trials have been conducted in this group of patients. Medications used are similar to those used for trigeminal neuralgia, with carbamazepine being the first-line agent. Other medications are described in chapter 11. These medications include anticonvulsants, antidepressants, and muscle relaxants. In patients with cardiac syncope, there has been a reported use of cardiac pacing. In patients who are unresponsive to medical management, procedural and surgical treatment may be needed.

If medications are ineffective, applying a local anesthetic to the back of the throat may provide temporary relief. Surgical options include nerve resection, tracheotomy, or microvascular decompression. However, there is little long-term follow-up with these cases.

PROGNOSIS

Spontaneous remission can occur in up to 75% of patients; therefore, some individuals recover from their initial attack and never have another. Others experience clusters of attacks followed by periods of short or long remission. Some individuals may have weight loss secondary to a fear that eating or drinking may cause an attack.

KEY POINTS TO REMEMBER

- Glossopharyngeal neuralgia is uncommon.
- GN is more common in men after the age of 40.
- There are secondary causes of GN; therefore, brain MRI is indicated.
- Medical treatment of GN is similar to that of trigeminal neuralgia, and is often focused on polypharmacy.
- Surgical options are available for patients who are refractory to medical management.

Further Reading

Carrieri PB, Montella S, Petracca M. Glossopharyngeal neuralgia as onset of multiple sclerosis. *Clin J Pain* 2009;25(8):737-739.

De Simone R, Ranieri A, Bilo L, Fiorillo C, Bonavita V. Cranial neuralgias: from physiopathology to pharmacological treatment. *Neurol Sci* May 2008; 29(Suppl 1):S69-78.

Ferroli P, Fioravanti A, Schiariti M, et al. Microvascular decompression for glossopharyngeal neuralgia: a long-term retrospectic review of the Milan-Bologna experience in 31 consecutive cases. *Acta Neurochir (Wien)* 2009;151(10):1245-1250.

Franzini A, Ferroli P, Messina G, Broggi G. Surgical treatment of cranial neuralgias. *Handb Clin Neurol* 97:679-692.

Kandan SR, Khan S, Jeyaretna DS, Lhatoo S, Patel NK, Coakham HB. Neuralgia of the glossopharyngeal and vagal nerves: long-term outcome following surgical treatment and literature review. *Br J Neurosurg* 2010;24(4):441-446.

McLaughlin MR, Jannetta PJ, Clyde BL, Subach BR, Comey CH, Resnick DK. Microvascular decompression of cranial nerves: lessons learned after 4400 operations. *J Neurosurg* 1999;90(1):1-8.

Resnick DK, Jannetta PJ, Bissonnette D, Jho HD, Lanzino G. Microvascular decompression for glossopharyngeal neuralgia. *Neurosurgery* 1995;36(1):64-68; discussion 68-69.

Rushton JG, Stevens JC, Miller RH. Glossopharyngeal (vagoglossopharyngeal) neuralgia: a study of 217 cases. *Arch Neurol* Apr 1981;38(4):201-205.

A 41-year-old male presents to the pain clinic with progressive onset of increased bilateral lower extremity burning pain and ongoing urinary hesitancy. He is 2 years status post lumbar spine surgery for herniated disc with initial symptom relief of low back pain and L5 radiculopathy. In the last year, however, he has developed constant pain and tingling in the lower extremity, increased with activity and improved with an anticonvulsant. He describes weakness in his legs and rated his pain as a 7/10 in severity.

He was recently reevaluated by his surgeon for his ongoing symptoms. Magnetic resonance imaging showed clumping of the lumbar nerve roots. Given the quality of his pain, his symptoms, and MRI findings, he was diagnosed with arachnoiditis and referred to the pain clinic for symptom management.

What do you do now?

This patient's diagnosis is arachnoiditis. Arachnoiditis describes a progressive pain disorder caused by the inflammation of the arachnoid, one of the membranes that surround and protect the nerves of the spinal cord and the subarachnoid space. Either the spinal cord and/or the brain may be involved. Since the subarachnoid space is continuous, it would be expected that a noxious agent introduced in one place would distribute itself throughout the space; however, such is not the case. Lumbar arachnoiditis is characterized by adherence of nerve roots to each other in the proximity of the cauda equina.

The arachnoid can become inflamed because of various causes.

- Injury-induced
  This is a rare complication of spinal surgery or trauma to the spine; may include advanced spinal stenosis, chronic compression of the spinal nerves, degenerative disc disease, or invasive procedures.

- Chemically induced
  In recent years, myelograms have been identified as a possible cause of this condition. A myelogram is a diagnostic test in which a radiographic contrast media is injected into the area surrounding the spinal cord and nerves to aid in diagnosis of various spinal conditions. There has been concern that exposure to these dyes, especially repeated exposure to oil-based dye, can precipitate arachnoiditis. In addition, there has been concern that epidural steroid injections may cause this condition, especially if the steroid medication enters the intrathecal space.

- Infection-induced
  Arachnoiditis may be caused by bacterial (syphilis, tuberculosis), fungal, or viral infections.

- Neoplastic
  The seeding of neoplastic cells in the cerebrospinal fluid, as well as hematogenous spread of systemic tumors has been cited as a rare cause of arachnoiditis.

SIGNS AND SYMPTOMS

Arachnoiditis is a progressive disease that can cause symptoms that are often debilitating and associated with disability. The condition is characterized by severe shooting pain of a stinging and burning quality that can be mild to severe and intractable. Depending on the location of the arachnoiditis, patients may have differing symptom location and neurologic sequelae. For example, the predominant symptom of lumbar arachnoiditis is pain in the lower back and lower extremities.

Arachnoiditis causes inflammation that can lead to the formation of scars and adhesions, which can cause the spinal nerves to coalesce and interfere with their function. This can result in the following symptoms:

- Tingling, numbness, or weakness and, in severe cases, paralysis
- Bizarre sensations such as insects crawling on the skin or water trickling down the leg.
- Muscle cramps, spasms, and twitching
- Bladder, bowel, and/or sexual dysfunction

DIAGNOSTIC CRITERIA

Arachnoiditis is clearly defined by pathologic and radiographic evidence. However, its clinical characteristics are eluding. Magnetic resonance is the imaging of choice for diagnosis; as in the "empty thecal sac sign," where the high contrast provided by the high cerebrospinal fluid signal on T2 weighted imaging identifies the clumped nerves of the disorder. MRI myelography may provide more information than MRI. Computed Tomography (CT) with myelogram identifies to a lesser degree the pathognomonic features of arachnoiditis, but is used in those patients who are unable to undergo MRI. A CT myelogram makes it possible to evaluate the neural tube as well as the appearance and location of the nerve roots, a basic CT only identifies nerve root calcification.

Arachnoiditis can also mimic the symptoms of other diseases, such as spinal cord tumors, cauda equina syndrome, arachnoiditis ossificans, and syringomyelia. These conditions should be excluded and treated accordingly.

MANAGEMENT

Arachnoiditis is a disorder that causes chronic pain and neurologic deficits and is difficult to treat because there is a lack of evidence-based therapeutic gold standards. In addition, the disorder has no predictable pattern or severity of symptoms and long-term outcomes are not reliable. Many patients with diagnosis of arachnoiditis also have underlying conditions that can cause similar symptoms, including spinal stenosis, disc herniations, and so forth.

The first treatment objective is to treat any primary pathology such as tumors, infections, or spinal pathology appropriately. If the clinical symptoms persist, treatment is focused on pain relief and symptom management.

Pharmacologic Treatment

Persistent arachnoiditis pain is treated in a fashion similar to neuropathic pain. Treatment consists of nonsteroidal anti-inflammatory drugs, corticosteroids, antispasm drugs, tricyclic antidepressants, anticonvulsants, and in some cases, opioids.

Nonpharmacologic Treatment

Treatment is focused on improving symptoms that impair daily function, therefore a regimen of physiotherapy, exercise, and psychotherapy is often recommended. Physical therapy and modalities such as hydrotherapy, massage, and hot/cold therapy are recommended to maintain muscle strength, range of motion, and mobility. Transcutaneous Electrical Nerve Stimulation (TENS) is a treatment in which a painless electrical current is sent to specific nerves through electrode patches that are placed on the skin. The mild electrical current generates heat that serves to relieve stiffness, improve mobility, and relieve pain.

Counseling, cognitive behavioral therapy, biofeedback, acupuncture, and hypnosis have been used for symptoms management, to improve patient function and quality of life.

Procedural and Surgical Treatment

Interventional treatment is controversial since the outcomes are generally poor and provide only short-term relief. Clinical trials of steroid are needed to determine the efficacy of these treatments.

In many cases, surgery is not recommended for arachnoiditis as it can cause more scar tissue to develop and expose the nerves to more trauma.

However, there are multiple surgical modalities that are utilized in patients with intractable pain, including neuroloysis, nerve grafting, and nerve transfer with little evidence to substantiate their efficacy. Spinal cord stimulation is proposed when intractable pain is the predominant symptom. It involves an implanted device that transmits an electrical signal to the dorsal column of the spinal cord for modulation of pain pathways and subsequent pain relief (see chapter 29).

KEY POINTS TO REMEMBER

- Arachnoiditis describes a progressive pain disorder caused by the inflammation of the arachnoid and characterized by adherence of nerve roots to each other.
- The arachnoid can become inflamed because of various causes; including injury, chemicals, infections, and neoplasms.
- MRI is the imaging of choice for diagnosis.
- There is a multimodal approach to treatment.

Further Reading

Di Ieva A, Barolat G, Tschabitscher M, et al. Lumbar arachnoiditis and thecaloscopy: brief review and proposed treatment algorithm. *Cen Eur Neurosurg* 2010;71(4):207-212.

Epter RS, Helm S 2nd, Hayek SM, Benyamin RM, Smith HS, Abdi S. Systematic review of percutaneous adhesiolysis and management of chronic low back pain in post lumbar surgery syndrome. *Pain Physician* 2009;12(2):361-378.

French JD. Clinical manifestations of lumbar spinal arachnoiditis. *Surgery* 1946;20(5): 718-729.

Nagayama M, Watanabe Y, Okumura A, Amoh Y, Nakashita S, Dodo Y. High-resolution single-slice MR myelography. *AJR Am J Roentgenol* 2002;179(2):515-521.

Nelson DA, Landau WM. Intraspinal steroids: history, efficacy, accidentality, and controversy with review of United States Food and Drug Administration reports. *J Neurol Neurosurg Psychiatry* 2001;70(4):433-443.

Petty PG, Hudgson P, Hare WS. Symptomatic lumbar spinal arachnoiditis: fact or fallacy? *J Clin Neurosci* 2000;7(5):395-399.

Shaw MD, Russell JA, Grossart KW. The changing pattern of spinal arachnoiditis. *J Neurol Neurosurg Psychiatry* 1978;41(2):97-107.

Wilkinson HA. Intrathecal depo-medrol: a literature review. *Clin J Pain* 1992;8(1):49-56; discussion 57-48.

Wright MH, Denney LC. A comprehensive review of spinal arachnoiditis. *Orthop Nurs* 2003;22(3):215-219; quiz 220-211.

Yang H, Wang R, Luo T, et al. MRI manifestations and differentiated diagnosis of postoperative spinal complications. *J Huazhong Univ Sci Technolog Med Sci* 2009;29(4):522-526.

18 Occipital Neuralgia

A 19-year-old male presents to the clinic with a 2-month history of headache, which started after hitting the back of his head against a shelf. The patient describes the pain as a continuous ache starting at the back of his head and radiating over the right side of his head to just behind his right eye. The pain is worse when laying on a pillow on the right side. The headache is associated with mild photophobia, scalp tenderness, and tenderness to palpation at the right upper cervical spine. He denies aura, phonophobia, loss of consciousness, or nausea and vomiting. Physical examination is notable for tenderness and hyperesthesia over the right occipital and parietal scalp. The patient also feels tenderness over the superior nuchal line midway between the mastoid and the occipital protuberance. Pain is worsened with extension of the neck. The remainder of his neurologic and musculoskeletal exam is normal.

What do you do now?

This patient is suffering from occipital neuralgia. Occipital neuralgia is defined by the International Headache Society (IHS) as paroxysmal shooting or stabbing pain in the dermatomes of the nervus occipitalis major or nervus occipitalis minor. There are very few reports on the prevalence and incidence of the disorder; however, as health care practitioners are becoming increasingly aware of the disorder, there are a greater number of referrals made to physicians who treat headache to help with diagnosing the problem.

The pain in occipital neuralgia is characterized as burning, lancinating pain that, like migraine, is usually unilateral with radiation to the frontal, orbital, and periorbital regions. The sensory changes can include hypo- or dysesthesia over these regions. Similarities between migraine and occipital neuralgia (ON) include scalp allodynia and occipital tenderness. Pain over the occipital nerve is usually pathognomonic for the diagnosis.

The causes of occipital neuralgia are many and varied and can be divided into four groups: vascular, neurogenic, muscular/tendinous, and osteogenic (Table 18.1). Ninety percent of the time the greater occipital nerve is the nerve involved, and 10% of the time it is the lesser occipital nerve.

TABLE 18.1 **Causes of Occipital Neuralgia**

Groups	Causes
Vascular	• Irritation of nerve roots at C1/C2 by an aberrant branch of PICA • Dural AV fistula at cervical level • Bulbocervical cavernoma bleeding • Cervical intramedullar cavernous hemangioma • Fenestrated vertebral artery pressing on C1/C2 nerve roots • Aberrant course of vertebral artery
Neurogenic	• Schwannoma at the craniocervical junction • C2 myelitis • Multiple sclerosis
Muscular/Tendinous	
Osteogenic	• C1/C2 arthrosis • Hypermobile posterior atlas • Cervical osteochondroma • Cranium osteolytic lesion • C1/C2 callus formation after fracture

DIAGNOSIS

Diagnosis is performed by taking a careful history, performing a physical exam, and continuing with any additional tests to help clarify the etiology of pain. History of occipital neuralgia will include complaints of shooting or stabbing pain in the neck radiating over the apex of the head. Patients may complain of pain in the back of the eye, vision impairment, tinnitus, dizziness, nausea, and nasal congestion.

Physical examination may demonstrate hypo- or dysesthesia over the areas innervated by the greater occipital nerve or lesser occipital nerve as well as tenderness to palpation over these areas. Local anesthetic blocks are used to help with the diagnosis.

Initial imaging with an X-ray of the cervical spine will be helpful for identifying any arthritis of the C2 facet joints or extruded callus formation after fracture. CT imaging can be useful for examining neoplastic or degenerative etiologies. MRI is very useful for evaluating cervical and occipital soft tissues, spinal cord, and nerve root pathologies.

TREATMENT

As with the treatment of most painful disorders, it is most prudent to start with conservative therapy. For the treatment of occipital neuralgia, this would include trial of therapy with attempts to improve cervical muscle tension, improve posture, and pharmacotherapy including tricyclic antidepressants, antiepileptics, and nonsteroidal anti-inflammatory agents.

Interventional management is now becoming a more common strategy for the management of occipital neuralgia. Interventional techniques include occipital nerve blocks with local anesthetic and corticosteroids; botulinum toxin A infiltration, which has evidence that is contradictory and is not commonly performed; pulsed radiofrequency treatment of the occipital nerve; and peripheral occipital nerve stimulation (see Figure 18.1).

When determining the flow of treatment, the following guidelines are most useful:

1. History and physical examination to determine the diagnosis of occipital neuralgia
2. Perform a test block to confirm diagnosis

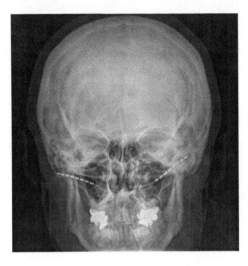

FIGURE 18.1 Radiographic imaging of patient with bilateral percutaneous leads placed along the occipital nerve in a patient suffering from occipital neuralgia. (Courtesy of Gilbert J. Fanciullo, MD, Department of Anesthesiology, Section of Pain Medicine, Dartmouth Hitchcock Medical Center, Lebanon, NH.)

3. Consider an occipital nerve block with local anesthetic and corticosteroid, or pulsed radiofrequency of the occipital nerve
4. If there is insufficient pain relief, consider occipital nerve stimulation

---

KEY POINTS TO REMEMBER

- Occipital neuralgia is defined by the International Headache Society (IHS) as paroxysmal shooting or stabbing pain in the dermatomes of the nervus occipitalis major or nervus occipitalis minor.
- Treatment flow guidelines start with history and physical exam, followed by performing a test block, then considering more long-term blocks with anesthetic and corticosteroid or with radiofrequency ablation of the occipital nerve.
- For refractory therapy, occipital nerve stimulation may be considered.

Further Reading

IHC IHSCS. International Classification of Headache Disorders: the international classification of headache disorders: 2nd edition. *Cephalalgia* 2004;24:1-160.

Sahai-Srivastava S, Zheng L. Occipital neuralgia with and without migraine: difference in pain characteristics and risk factors. *Headache* 2011;51:124-128.

Vaneldren P, Lataster A, Levy R, et al. Evidence-based medicine: evidence-based interventional pain medicine according to Clinical Diagnoses chapter 8. Occipital Neuralgia. *Pain Pract* 2010;10:137-144.

19 Cancer Pain

A 52-year-old woman presents with a 3-month history of tingling in her left shoulder, forearm, and hand. The tingling, which began 3 months ago, has been gradually increasing in intensity to the point where for the past 2 weeks she has had a burning pain in her shoulder and notices clumsiness of her hand. She relates a past medical history of breast cancer in the left breast with lumpectomy, axial node dissection, radiation, and chemotherapy for treatment when she was 40 years old. There has been no evidence of recurrence, and she considers herself completely cured.

On physical examination, she has allodynia over the deltoid and hypesthesia to pinprick and fine touch in the hand and forearm in a distribution not isolating a particular nerve. She has mild, diffuse weakness from a C5 to a C8 distribution in that arm. Her history, review of systems, and physical examination is otherwise entirely normal. A thorough recent evaluation by her oncologist showed no evidence of tumor recurrence. Electromyography shows myokymic discharges and axonal motor and sensory neuropathy in the area described.

What do you do now?

mproved cancer therapy has led to increasing life expectancy and cure rates in most types of cancer. The American Cancer Society has stated a goal of making cancer into a chronic disease state in which long-term control is possible even in the absence of a conventional cure. There are 10 million cancer survivors in the United States alone; 1.4 million Americans were newly diagnosed with cancer in 2004. This is approximately 4,000 patients per day. In that same year, 564,000 patients died from cancer. Approximately 3% of the population of the United States is currently living with cancer.

Posttreatment pain syndromes can stem from chemotherapy, radiation, or surgery. Postchemotherapy painful peripheral neuropathy is well described with the use of a variety of agents. Radiation-induced neural damage and pain may present decades after radiotherapy completion, often confounding the diagnosis. Postsurgical pain syndromes come in many varieties including post mastectomy, post amputation, post thoracotomy, and a variety of other chronic pain conditions.

The prevalence of chronic pain in breast cancer survivors is estimated to be 50%. The types of pain that occur can be complex, difficult to diagnosis, may be myalgic or neuropathic, and might be less responsive than other pain syndromes to usual treatments. Radiation-induced plexopathy may occur up to 20 years after cancer treatment. Pain in breast cancer survivors may present in the arm, neck, shoulder, axilla, chest wall, or breast. Paresthesia, dysesthesia, allodynia, hyperalgesia, and loss of shoulder function have all been reported. Many providers believe that breast-conserving treatment results in a decreased incidence of chronic pain, but this has not been shown to be a fact; and in fact, there is evidence that breast-conserving surgery with axillary node dissection may result in a higher incidence of chronic pain than radical mastectomy. This is likely related to the increased use of chemotherapy and radiotherapy in patients having more-conservative resections. There is also some evidence that women who have a breast prosthesis may have a higher incidence of chronic pain.

The best predictor of chronic pain in breast cancer survivors is likely the severity of acute postoperative pain. This may be related to the prevalence of underrecognized neuropathic pain, and less-skilled postoperative management. It may also be related to the high prevalence of depression and anxiety in patients undergoing surgery, surgical technique (for example, traction), and postoperative complications such as bleeding or infection. Postoperative radiation therapy is a risk factor for pain in both the breast and the arm. Preemptive use of antineuropathic pain medications such as gabapentin may have a role in reducing the incidence of chronic pain.

Late effects of radiotherapy, which can include connective tissue fibrosis, neural damage, or secondary malignancies, can occur decades after completion of radiotherapy; and the incidence of mild plexopathy in women undergoing radiation therapy for breast cancer has been estimated to be as high as 9% with disabling, painful plexopathy estimates hovering in the 1-to-5% range. There is no specific, clinical presentation of radiation-induced plexopathy that can distinguish this syndrome from tumor recurrence other than the fact that tumor recurrence tends to involve the lower trunks of the plexus and may present in an ulnar distribution, whereas radiation tends to involve C5, 6, or 7 roots. Nerve conduction studies can be normal in 10% of patients with radiation-induced brachial plexopathy. It is not uncommon for radiation-induced plexopathy to progress to a flaccid arm. In one study of 33 patients with radiation-induced brachial plexopathy, the authors reported 17 patients required opioids for treatment of their pain, and once onset of plexopathy occurred, progression was inexorable and led to loss of useful hand function in a time range of between 6 weeks and 5 years.

Psychological factors influence chronic pain in patients cured of cancer. Patients are afraid to report their pain because they are afraid it may indicate a recurrence of their tumor. Patients who use active coping strategies report less chronic pain than those who use passive strategies; catastrophizing is common. Early institution of behavioral medicine strategies in the treatment of both acute and chronic cancer pain may result in an improved quality of life for survivors. Physical therapy can be extremely useful.

The same interdisciplinary treatment paradigms apply to cancer survivors as apply to all chronic pain patients. The proper balance of interventional treatments, pharmacological treatments, behavioral interventions, and physical medicine approaches will produce the best outcome. Pharmacological management should be mechanism based, and with a neuropathic syndrome such as in the patient described, antineuropathic pain medication paradigms should be followed.

- There are more than 10 million cancer survivors in the United States, and the prevalence of chronic pain in subsets of this population may be as high as 50%.

- Chronic pain after cancer is usually related to treatment and is more common when treatment combinations such as surgery plus chemotherapy plus radiation therapy are utilized.

- Pain syndromes secondary to radiation therapy may not occur for up to 20 years after treatment.

- Radiation-induced brachial plexopathy often progresses to complete loss of function of the arm and requires opioids to help manage the pain.

Further Reading

Fanciullo GJ, Beasley R. Chronic pain in the cured cancer patient. In: *Cancer Pain Management* (Fisch MJ, Burton AW, eds), 2007, pp 189-198, McGraw Hill Medical, New York.

Perkins FM, Kehlet H. Chronic pain as an outcome of surgery: a review of predictive factors. *Anesthesiology* 2000;93:1123-1133.

20 Mononeuropathy

A 56-year-old male with known type II diabetes mellitus presents to the pain clinic with pain along the left lateral thigh without evidence of back or hip pain. He states that the pain is lancinating and burning in character and associated with a pins and needles sensation in his left lateral thigh. Diagnostic studies show an HbA1c of 12 and blood glucose of 300, and MRI of the lumbar spine does not indicate any significant abnormalities. A fascicular biopsy of the nerve in the lateral thigh shows small diameter regenerating myelinated fibers and evidence of diabetic microangiopathy.

What do you do now?

M ononeuropathies are a not uncommon source of pain, of which one of the most notable is postherpetic neuralgia, which is covered in chapter 3. Other notable painful mononeuropathies include diabetic mononeuropathy and amyotrophy, mononeuropathy multiplex, entrapment neuropathies, and mononeuropathies due to peripheral nerve tumors.

TYPES OF MONONEUROPATHIES

Diabetic Mononeuropathy and Amyotrophy

Mononeuropathy is a nerve injury that specifically targets one nerve, and thus the symptoms exhibited correspond to the anatomical function of the nerve that was injured. Compared to the normal population, diabetic patients have an increased predisposition to mononeuropathies, of which mononeuropathies of the motor nerves serving extraocular movements, as well as of the peripheral nerves, are the most common in location. Painful mononeuropathies of the cranial nerves responsible for extraocular movements can manifest days prior to the onset of actual muscle weakness, and are characterized as pain starting behind or around the eye. Mononeuropathies can also extend to the periphery as well as the thoracic nerves specifically targeting the median, ulnar, peroneal, femoral, and lateral cutaneous nerves. As with the nerves of extraocular movement, pain is a common symptom of peripheral nerve mononeuropathy.

Another painful diabetic proximal neuropathy is termed diabetic amyotrophy. Diabetic amyotrophy is now more commonly termed either proximal diabetic neuropathy or lumbosacral radiculoplexus neuropathy and described as painful proximal muscle wasting and weakness. Presentation is usually asymmetric, and there is usually a loss of normal patellar reflexes on the side that is affected. EMG can be performed and will show evidence of a mixed axonal and demyelinating neuropathy affecting the proximal musculature. The pathology is thought to be due to microangiopathic changes causing ischemia to the peripheral nerves.

Mononeuritis Multiplex

Mononeuritis multiplex is a disease state characterized by multiple noncontiguous mononeuropathies occurring acutely to chronically over months to many years that presents with loss of sensory or motor function of individual

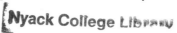

peripheral nerves. This type of neuropathy is often associated with pain that is neuropathic in quality, and is also characterized as deep, aching pain, worse at night, and located mostly in the back, hip, and thigh. EMG can be done to examine the patient and will show signs consistent with multifocal sensory motor axonal neuropathy.

Commonly associated systemic illnesses include diabetes mellitus, vasculitides, autoimmune disease including SLE and sarcoidosis, leprosy, Lyme disease, HIV infection, amyloidosis, cryoglobulinemia, and chemical agents.

Entrapment Neuropathies

Entrapment neuropathies are most commonly due to compression of nerves traversing narrow passages. Most common locations include the carpal tunnel and spinal roots exiting the foramen due to compression by adjacent herniated discs or hypertrophy of the associated facet joint. This usually results in a painful condition that may be associated with paresthesias, muscle weakness, and numbness along the pathway of the nerve affected. The underlying pathophysiology indicates that entrapment leads to damage and reduction of the myelinated fibers with persistence of the C-fibers. This is thought to be due to microangiopathic changes leading to ischemia of the larger myelinated fibers. Patients will describe the pain as burning, pins and needles, and lancinating pain. EMG in early disease may not show evidence of demyelination of the larger nerves, and does not do a particularly good job of describing pathology of the C-fibers.

There are many examples of entrapment neuropathies, including carpal tunnel syndrome, Morton's neuralgia, and radiculopathy. Morton's neuralgia is due to severe entrapment of the plantar digital nerve on the metatarsal heads of the foot. Patients will complain of burning pain at the bottom of their foot and at the bottom of their toe.

Proper history and physical, as well as EMG are the diagnostic tools of choice. MRI of the spine may be helpful for showing structural abnormalities including herniated discs and facet hypertrophy as a cause of spinal nerve root compression. For those with pain associated with thoracic outlet syndrome, MRI is again the diagnostic test of choice to examine structures that may be compressing the exiting brachial plexus causing severe pain in the upper shoulder.

Peripheral Nerve Tumors

Peripheral nerve tumors are a rare source of painful mononeuropathy but must be included in the differential when evaluating a patient with mononeuropathy. Tumors associated are commonly benign schwannomas, neurofibromas, neurinomas, and less commonly, malignant neuromas. Presenting symptoms may include local tenderness, paresthesias in the distribution of the affected nerve, swelling, pain, and palpable masses for those that are more superficially located. The diagnostic modality of choice for those that may be deeper is MRI with contrast. Tissue biopsy should be performed for histologic characterization of the mass.

MANAGEMENT

The best treatment for the aforementioned disease states is careful treatment of the underlying source, which can include tight control of blood glucose, treatment of infectious causes with antibiotics or antivirals, and so forth. Medical therapy utilizing anticonvulsants and antidepressants may be useful in targeting the neuropathic pain components. As well, topical anesthetics may be used for symptoms of allodynia and dysesthesia. As a last resort, if all other therapies do not appear helpful, spinal cord stimulation may prove to be useful in decreasing pain.

KEY POINTS TO REMEMBER

- Mononeuropathies are a not uncommon source of pain, of which one of the most notable is postherpetic neuralgia, which is covered in its own section of this book.
- Other notable painful mononeuropathies include diabetic mononeuropathy and amyotrophy, mononeuropathy multiplex, entrapment neuropathies, and mononeuropathies due to peripheral nerve tumors.
- Diagnosis is via EMG, MRI, and tissue biopsy in some cases.
- Treatment is aimed at treating the underlying disorder and palliation with oral anticonvulsants or antidepressants.

Further Reading

Dyck PJ, Thomas PK. *Diabetic Neuropathy.* Saunders, Philadelphia,1999.

Dyck PJ, Thomas PK. *Peripheral Neuropathy.* Saunders, Philadelphia, 2005.

Heck AW, Phillips LH 2nd. Sarcoidosis and the nervous system. *Neurol Clin* 1989;7(3): 641–654.

Said G, Lacroix C, Lozeron P, et al. Inflammatory vasculopathy in multifocal diabetic neuropathy. *Brain* 2003;126:376–385.

Chronic Pain and Related Disorders

21 Chronic Pain and Depression

A 33-year-old female presents to her primary care provider's office with a 5-year history of chronic low back pain. She describes a constant, aching pain that radiates from her low back into her buttock with a pain level of 8 out of 10. She has been evaluated by multiple providers and has been involved in physical therapy as well as medical management, and is not a candidate for any surgical approach to her pain.

She continues to suffer from pain, which is limiting her quality of life. She had worked as a dental receptionist, however secondary to pain, she has quit her job and is caring for her two children at home. She is very discouraged that she continues to suffer from pain and feels as if no treatment modalities are helping with her symptoms. She has a personal history of childhood physical abuse and describes feeling depressed most days, which she relates only to the fact that she has pain. In addition, she suffers from sleep dysfunction and poor appetite. On further discussion, the patient feels as if her condition is hopeless and asserts that if her physicians had treatment that would decrease her pain, her depression would be controlled. At this time, she is unwilling to see a therapist and refuses antidepressants, as she believes she has pain and not depression.

What do you do now?

This patient is suffering from chronic pain, as well as depression. According to the International Association for the Study of Pain (IASP), the definition of pain is "an unpleasant sensory and emotional experience associated with actual or potential tissue damage, or described in terms of such damage." Chronic pain is a complex experience that affects a patient's thoughts, mood, and behavior. Based on this, it resembles depression, and the relationship between depression and pain is linked. The studies of patients with chronic pain show that up to 90% have axis I disorders and up to 59% have axis II disorders. Chronic pain is associated with considerable psychopathology, and treatment should be focused on a multimodal approach.

The convergence of depression and pain is reflected in our biological system. In the nervous system, brain pathways handle the reception of pain signals including the emotions and limbic system, as well as divert signals of physical discomfort so that we can concentrate on the external milieu. When this is impaired, physical sensations, including pain, can be more central in the patient's perceptions. Similar neurotransmitters are involved in the regulation of mood and in pain reception, especially serotonin and norepinephrine. When regulation of these pathways fails, pain can intensify and mood can be depressed.

HOW DEPRESSION AND PAIN AFFECT DISABILITY

Depression contributes to the disability caused by chronic pain conditions including back pain, headache, abdominal pain, or arthritis. Patients in pain who are depressed become heavy consumers of medical services, even when no significant pathology is identified.

Published data regarding major depression as a comorbidity factor in patients with chronic pain gives prevalence rates between 1.5 and 57% and even as high as 72%. It is well established that depression occurs more often in individuals with pain for a range of physical disorders. Kroenke and Price (1993) demonstrated that any physical symptoms increased the likelihood of depression in 34% of patients with joint and limb pain, 40% with headaches, 46% with chest pain, and 43% with abdominal pain. It appears, therefore, that depression is more likely to occur in physical illnesses or after injuries if chronic pain is present. In addition, when depression is present, it is associated with increased functional impairment.

MANAGEMENT

Patients who present to primary care offices and to other clinicians with chronic pain and depression are frequently undiagnosed or undertreated. In most visits, pain symptoms take center stage. The result is depression along with symptoms of appetite suppression, energy loss, sleep disturbance, and decreased physical activity, all of which confound the patient's pain. Therefore, as there is a connection between chronic pain and depression, it makes sense that treatment for these conditions will overlap.

Pharmacologic Treatment

Because chronic pain and depression involve similar neurotransmitters, antidepressants are used to treat both conditions. These medications act in brain pathways to reduce the perception of pain and regulate mood. The two major types of antidepressants that are used are the tricyclics and selective serotonin reuptake inhibitors (SSRIs). In addition, a newer antidepressant that works strongly on both neurotransmitters is believed to be superior for treating pain (serotonin norepinephrine reuptake inhibitors or SNRIs), however, the evidence is inconclusive. These medications are often started to help to improve patients' mood and decrease their pain (see Table 25.1).

Nonpharmacologic Treatment

Physical Activity

There are a good proportion of patients with chronic pain who avoid exercise, as they believe they have an increased risk of injury and worse pain with activity. Each patient should be evaluated individually; however, a well-designed exercise plan should be formulated, as exercise can decrease symptoms of depression. Physical therapists can provide exercises to help to decrease pain and improve mobility.

Psychological Treatment

Cognitive and behavioral therapies can teach chronic pain patients how to decrease avoidance behavior, including fearful anticipation, discouraging thoughts, and assist in addressing routines to decrease physical and emotional suffering and improve quality of life. Patients should be referred to cognitive behavioral therapists and psychotherapy to help with their symptoms.

Procedural and Surgical Treatment

Along with treating patients through medications and physical and psychological modalities, some patients may benefit from procedural therapy for their chronic pain. In addition, surgical treatment may be an option for some patients who may show pathology amendable to these modalities.

CONCLUSION

In treating patients with chronic pain with a comorbidity of depression, the focus is on a multimodal approach to their treatment including medications in the form of antidepressants, anti-inflammatories, occasional opioids, physical medicine, psychological medicine, and procedural therapy if applicable.

KEY POINTS TO REMEMBER

- Chronic pain is a complex experience.
- Similar neurotransmitters are involved in the regulation of mood and in pain reception; especially serotonin and norepinephrine
- Antidepressants act in brain pathways to reduce the perception of pain and regulate mood.
- Patients should be referred to cognitive behavioral therapists and psychotherapy to help with their symptoms.

Further Reading

Fishbain DA, Cutler R, Rosomoff HL, Rosomoff RS. Chronic pain-associated depression: antecedent or consequence of chronic pain? A review. *Clin J Pain* 1997;13(2):116-137.

Fishbain DA, Goldberg M, Meagher BR, Steele R, Rosomoff H. Male and female chronic pain patients categorized by DSM-III psychiatric diagnostic criteria. *Pain* 1986;26(2):181-197.

Gallagher RM, Moore P, Chernoff I. The reliability of depression diagnosis in chronic low back pain: a pilot study. *Gen Hosp Psychiatry* 1995;17(6):399-413.

Goldenberg D, Mayskiy M, Mossey C, Ruthazer R, Schmid C. A randomized, double-blind crossover trial of fluoxetine and amitriptyline in the treatment of fibromyalgia. *Arthritis Rheum* 1996;39(11):1852-1859.

Kroenke K, Price RK. Symptoms in the community: prevalence, classification, and psychiatric comorbidity. *Arch Intern Med* 8 1993;153(21):2474-2480.

Large RG. DSM-III diagnoses in chronic pain: confusion or clarity? *J Nerv Ment Dis* 1986;174(5):295-303.

Woerz R. Pain in depression–depression in pain. *Pain* 2003;Clinical Updates X(5).

22 Chronic Pain and Addictive Disorder

A 27-year-old woman presents with severe chronic chest wall and knee pain. She was diagnosed with sickle-cell disease when she was 12 years old and has had recurrent hospitalizations and crises every since. She is typically admitted to the hospital six or seven times a year with painful crises and suffers from avascular necrosis and a chest wall syndrome resulting in episodes of pneumonia at least yearly for the past 3 years.

She is disabled and unable to work and has exhibited multiple behaviors over the years consistent with pseudo-addiction and ultimately she was diagnosed with opioid addiction. She suffers from depression and anxiety with multiple attempts aimed at treatment in the past but refractory largely due to noncompliance. She has an erratic and stressful social situation, living with persons who will steal her drugs and supply her with other drugs. Her environment at times has been violent, and she has been a victim of physical abuse. She continues to smoke one pack of cigarettes per day and has been incarcerated in the past for drug-related infractions. She is referred to you by her primary care provider, who has been prescribing methadone 10 mg three times a day to her, along with oxycodone/acetaminophen 10 mg/325 mg three times a day as needed. Her primary care provider is committed to her care, but needs advice and support for continued management.

What do you do now?

The American Society of Addiction Medicine has defined addiction as a primary chronic disease of brain reward, motivation, memory, and related circuitry. Dysfunction of these circuits leads to characteristic, biological, psychological, social, and spiritual manifestations. This is reflected in the individual pursuing reward and/or relief by substance use and other behaviors. The addiction is characterized by impairment in behavioral control, craving, inability to consistently abstain, and diminished recognition of significant problems with one's behaviors and interpersonal relationships. Like other chronic diseases, addiction involves cycles of relapse and remission. Without treatment or engagement in recovery activities, addiction is progressive and can result in disability or premature death.

Risk stratification for this patient includes consideration of evidence of an objective painful disorder, family history, personal history, employment, and behavior. This patient clearly suffers from the disease addiction and confounding this diagnosis is the fact that she clearly suffers from a severe and painful disease, which if not treated appropriately with analgesics, can result in hospitalization and premature death.

Patients with refractory noncompliance and abuse issues are at high risk for harming themselves due to their behaviors, and providers prescribing opioids to them may be at high-risk for feelings of insecurity and guilt, as well as medical/legal consequences if the patients harm themselves or others with their prescriptions. High-risk patients may be managed by a committed provider with intensive educational support, the use of a multidisciplinary team including an addiction specialist, frequent visits—perhaps at times even weekly—for prescriptions, and urine toxicology monitoring to at least understand what other drugs the patients may be using and/or compliance.

A national survey on drug use conducted by the Substance Abuse and Mental Health Services Administration showed that the drug categories with the largest number of recent initiatives among persons aged 12 or older were the nonmedical use of pain relievers (2.176 million) and marijuana (2.208 million). In 2008, the number of new nonmedical users of oxycontin, aged 12 and over was 478,000, with an average age at first use of 22.6 years. Persons abusing these drugs are more likely to be males, unemployed, or patients with a history of incarceration. The rate of abuse in patients on parole is more than 25% compared to an average population rate of abuse of approximately 8%. The source of prescription drugs among persons 12 years of age or older was most commonly, 60% of the time, obtained from a friend or relative for free. Approximately 9% bought the drug from a friend or a relative, and 5% took them from a friend or relative without asking. Eighteen percent reportedly got the drugs from a doctor. Only 4.3% reported receiving their pain relievers from a drug dealer or a stranger.

The therapeutic use of opioids in the United States has exploded, with increased sales of hydrocodone of almost 300% from 1997 to 2007, increased use of methadone of almost 1300%, and oxycodone of almost 900%. In 2003, there were 354 million prescriptions for opioids written in the United States. The Drug Abuse Warning Network reported almost 90,000 emergency room visits associated with the use of hydrocodone in 2008, and over 105,000 oxycodone visits. Unintentional overdose deaths are much higher for opioid analgesics than for either cocaine or heroin, and in 2007 there were almost 28,000 unintentional drug overdose deaths in the United States. These were second only to motor vehicle crash deaths, and in many states in the United States with more recent data, the deaths related to prescription opioid abuse now exceed the deaths related to motor vehicle accidents.

Opioids at the same time are one of the most useful drugs in a physician's armamentaria. Good pain management utilizing a multiple pharmacological approach along with behavioral medicine and physical medicine approaches might prevent hospitalizations, episodes of pneumonia or other infections, and possibly prolong life in a patient such as the one we have described. Unfortunately the potential harm to providers, our patient, ourself, society, and payers, make it virtually impossible, in the case of intractable abuse, to manage this patient with opioids. This patient, however, is not without options, and it may be that treatment with buprenorphine or methadone could be useful not only to manage her pain but also to manage her opioid addiction. Buprenorphine is an opioid agonist that is approximately 30 times as potent as morphine, and joint management between an addictionologist and pain medicine specialist or a provider with a special interest and special skill in pain medicine, might be able to successfully manage this patient. The thing to do next would not be to continue to prescribe relatively low doses of methadone and as needed oxycodone, but to find an addictionologist who can help comanage her with methadone or buprenorphine.

CONCLUSION

The management of patients with both addictive disorder and chronic pain can lead to frustration and feelings of uncertainty for providers. Patients with severe painful disease deserve to be treated with opioids but must also be protected from harm.

KEY POINTS TO REMEMBER

- Addiction is characterized by impairment in behavioral control, craving, inability to consistently abstain, and diminished recognition of significant problems with one's behaviors and interpersonal relationships.
- High-risk patients should be managed by a committed provider and should involve intensive educational support, the use of a multidisciplinary team including an addiction specialist, frequent visits for prescriptions, and urine toxicology monitoring.

Further Reading

Gilson AM. State medical board members' attitudes about the legality of chronic prescribing to patients with noncancer pain: the influence of knowledge and beliefs about pain management, addiction, and opioid prescribing. J Pain Sympt Manage 2010;40(4):599-612.

Markowitz JD, Francis EM, Gonzales-Nolas C. Managing acute and chronic pain in a substance abuse treatment program for the addicted individual early in recovery: a current controversy. J Psychoactive Drugs 2010;42(2):193-198.

Walwyn WM, Miotto KA, Evans CJ. Opioid pharmaceuticals and addiction: the issues, and research directions seeking solutions. Drug Alcohol Depend 2010;108(3):156-165.

Webster LR, Fine PG. Approaches to improve pain relief while minimizing opioid abuse liability. J Pain 2010;11(7):602-611.

23 Chronic Pain And Other Psychiatric Disorders

A 62-year-old male with a history of diffuse aches and pains that are nonspecific in location presents to the clinic to discuss possible treatment options to help relieve his pain. The patient appears restless on presentation, often holding different parts of his body and grimacing in pain, makes poor eye contact, and has pressured, goal-directed speech. When asked about the onset of symptoms he states that they happened sometime after his return from the Korean War but associated the pain with multiple injuries encountered during the war. He has been tried on multiple antidepressants, anticonvulsants, opiates, and nonsteroidal medications without relief. He states that the pain wakes him from sleep at night and he often has flashbacks to the Korean War with increased startle response.

What do you do now?

The patient is suffering from chronic pain with associated psychiatric comorbidity.

ANXIETY DISORDERS

The anxiety disorders are a common set of psychiatric disorders affecting not only those with chronic pain, but also the general population. The experience of anxiety is a common universal emotion. However, painful acute or chronic illnesses can bring on a sense of anxiety not only with learning how to interpret pain (i.e., the concept of hurt versus harm), but also in coping with the frustrations of treatment effects, prolonged or changing symptomatology, and those effects on the daily life of the individual dealing with the illness. The point at which this sense of anxiety becomes pathologic is when the anxiety becomes incapacitating.

Post-Traumatic Stress Disorder

Post-traumatic stress disorder (PTSD) is defined as the presence of symptoms greater than 1 month and that cause impairment in functioning associated with the following:

1. Exposure to a traumatic event in which the person experienced or witnessed events that resulted in or threatened death, or serious injury, or a threat to the physical integrity of self or others, AND the person felt fear, helplessness, or horror.
2. "Reexperiencing" by recurrence of one of the following: intrusive thoughts, distressing dreams of the event, reliving the event (dissociative flashbacks, hallucinations, etc.), intense distress related to internal or external cues of the event, physiological reactivity related to internal or external cues of the event.
3. Avoidance of reminders, avoiding talking or thinking about the event, detachment from others, restricted range of affect, foreshortened future, can't remember parts of the event, reduced interest in activities.
4. Increased arousal such as problems with sleep, irritability, concentration, hypervigilance, exaggerated startle.

The prevalence of PTSD in the general population is estimated to be 7–12%, while in the chronic pain population is estimated at 10–50%.

It is thought that the cognitive, affective, and behavioral components of chronic pain may exacerbate and maintain the symptoms of and responses to PTSD. An attentional bias toward pain related stimuli may amplify pain perception. Also, pain may be a reminder of the trauma and trigger arousal, thus escalating both PTSD symptoms and pain. The Mutual Maintenance Model to explain pain and PTSD includes four points:

1. Attentional biases may be present in chronic pain and PTSD patients such that they attend to threatening or painful stimuli.
2. Anxiety sensitivity may contribute toward a vulnerability to catastrophize.
3. Pain may be a reminder of the traumatic event, triggering an arousal response, avoidance of the cause of pain, and any memories of the trauma.
4. In both disorders, avoidance is used to minimize pain and disturbing thoughts.
5. Fatigue and lethargy associated with depression may contribute to both disorders.
6. General anxiety may contribute to both disorders.
7. Cognitive demands from symptoms of pain and PTSD limit the use of adaptive coping strategies.

The most common treatment strategy for PTSD is exposure therapy, which can be coupled with paroxetine or setraline, which are the two medications that are FDA approved for PTSD.

SOMATOFORM DISORDERS

Pain Disorder

The DSM IV-TR criteria for pain disorder state that pain at one or more sites forms the basis and that psychological factors are judged to be important in the onset, severity, exacerbations, or maintenance of the pain. The pain should cause significant distress and/or impaired function that cannot be better accounted for by a mood, anxiety, or a psychotic disorder. If a general medical condition is considered to be a cause at the onset of the painful condition, or in the severity, exacerbations, or maintenance, then pain disorder as a diagnosis should not be entertained. Also, if the condition is intentionally produced, then this should raise the concern for malingering.

Patients who present with pain disorder should still undergo a thorough workup, including a careful physical examination as well as examination of their mental health. This diagnosis is one of exclusion, and all other organic pathologies should be discounted first as the source for the onset, severity, exacerbations, or maintenance of the painful disorder.

Hypochondriasis

The definition of hypochondriacal disorder is the preoccupation by the individual of their health in the absence of an obvious cause for anxiety. The individual fails to respond to reassurance by medical providers, even after all studies performed have been completed. When the symptoms are treated, there is a short-lived improvement and then the patient will usually return with recurrent symptoms.

Some patients may even acknowledge that their anxieties are excessive; however, the preoccupation still drives them to continuously seek reassurance or further testing. It is not uncommon for the site of preoccupation to move, thus, a patient's history will often reveal multiple sites of symptom complaints. Patients are best treated with reassurance and treatment of any underlying anxiety or depression. Clinicians should avoid reinforcing the condition by doing unnecessary investigations and treatments. Cognitive behavioral therapy has also been proven useful for the treatment of this disorder.

Somatization Disorder

The DSM-IV criteria for somatization disorder include:

1. A history of four or more pain symptoms occurring in four or more different sites, including pain during menstruation or sexual intercourse.
2. Two gastrointestinal symptoms other than pain, i.e., nausea, vomiting, diarrhea, constipation, etc.
3. One sexual symptom, or symptoms related to the reproductive system other than pain, i.e., sexual indifference, erectile or ejaculatory dysfunction, etc.
4. One pseduoneurological symptom suggesting a neurological condition but not limited to pain, i.e., paralysis, loss of speech, loss of hearing, etc.

The symptoms must not be intentionally produced or feigned. The disorder must result in significant social, occupational, or other impairment. When physical examinations and other forms of testing are done, there are no organic causes to support the multiple complaints. Also, the complaints cannot be explained by substance abuse. Those patients who suffer from somatization disorder, often have significant comorbid depression and/or anxiety.

Conversion Disorder
Conversion disorder is used to describe a condition in which an individual develops paralysis, loss of hearing, visual loss, or memory loss due to severe underlying psychological disturbance. Those who suffer from conversion disorder are thought to be using the physical symptoms to avoid the emotional conflict that underlies. The connection between the stress and the physical symptoms is not appreciated by the individual. This, in turn, may relieve the person from any responsibilities at work and other activities, which is considered a "secondary" gain.

Personality Disorders
It has been estimated that up to 50% of patients with chronic low back pain were found to have at least one personality disorder. The most common types were antisocial, borderline, and paranoid personality disorders. When present, these portend a poor prognosis to recovery from chronic pain. As well, pain tends to intensify in terms of severity when there is a comorbid personality disorder.

KEY POINTS TO REMEMBER
- Chronic pain patients often present with a comorbid psychiatric abnormality, of which the anxiety disorders and depression are the most common.
- Concomitant treatment of the psychiatric disorder not only improves emotional health, but can also improve pain scores, functional improvement, and overall sense of well-being.
- Treatment with antidepressants and with psychiatric therapy is the mainstay of treatment.

Further Reading

Benedikt RA, Kolb LC. Preliminary findings on chronic pain and post-traumatic stress disorder. *Am J Psychiatry* 1986;143:908–910.

Polatin PB, Kinney RK, Gatchel RA, et al. Psychiatric illness behaviour. *Br J Med Psychol* 1993;51:131–137.

Sharp TJ, Harvey AG. Chronic pain and posttraumatic stress disorder: mutual maintenance? *Clin Psychol Rev* 2001;21:857–877.

24 The Difficult Chronic Pain Patient

A 42-year-old disabled professor of psychology presents with a 5-year history of diffuse body pains. She states that she has been diagnosed with fibromyalgia, is extremely knowledgeable about this illness, the literature surrounding fibromyalgia, and all the treatment options. She states that she was previously a patient of the provider's colleague from a nearby city, but had to dissolve that relationship because he was unable to provide the care that she needed. She had a 4-inch-thick pile of medical records from various institutions including the Mayo Clinic and Massachusetts General Hospital where she had been seen, and what she considered to be seminal articles addressing fibromyalgia.

She had previously read about the provider's accomplishments on the Internet and was delighted to be seeing such an excellent doctor. She was being treated with optimal doses of pregabalin and milnacipran and was using methadone 15 mg three times a day. She had no relief from nonsteroidal anti-inflammatory drugs; was unable to exercise at all because her pain was worsened by any physical activity; and saw no need to see a behavioral medicine specialist or mental health specialist because of her own previous training. She denied depression or anxiety and stated that she had never been treated for any mental health illnesses in the past. She declined to comment on a prior history of physical or sexual abuse.

She was accompanied by her husband, who was quiet and reading a book during the entire visit. She had a negative CAGE and a negative Screener for Opioid Abuse in Pain Patients and denies having ever had a problem with alcoholism or drug abuse. She did not know who her parents were because she was adopted, and she had multiple major stressors ongoing. She stated that her younger brother had recently committed suicide and that her mother was in the hospital with a stroke. She was here because she felt her methadone was not working as well as it used to and wished to inquire about either an increase in her dose or a rotation to a different drug. Her speech was loud and aggressive and she often veered off on tangents and could not be redirected. When attempts at redirecting the interview were made, she increased her volume and intensity of speech and made a somewhat threatening face and persisted in her discourse. She stated that because of her education, training, and depth of knowledge on the subject of fibromyalgia, she often required more time than other patients with her provider. She wished for the provider to take over her prescribing for all of her pain medications and to see her on a regular basis.

During the interview the provider felt clear negative feelings toward this patient, which included frustration and a clear sense of dislike. An opioid rotation resulted in daily phone calls. She declined to speak to the nurses in the clinic and instead insisted on speaking to the provider. When seen in the office a month later, she had no relief from her rotation and wished to go back on the methadone, but at a higher dose, as she had originally requested. When again advised that the provider would not increase the dose, she loudly began instructing the provider about opioid treatment for chronic pain, and again exceeded her scheduled appointment time. She persisted in calling the clinic every couple of days and when advised that the provider would no longer speak to her on the phone unless it were a medical emergency, had regular conversations with the nurses that often lasted 30 minutes. Her monthly visits with the provider continued to be aggressive, demanding, rude, and ultimately threatening. She threatened to report me to the Board of Medicine for my poor care. At this point, she was informed that the provider would no longer be able to care of her and that she should find another provider for her prescriptions. The provider also called her previous provider at this point, who related a similar experience treating this patient and expressed tremendous gratitude for having taken her off his hands.

What do you do now?

It has been estimated that one quarter of patients treated by physicians, nurses, and physician assistants exhibit "difficult behavior." The percentage of patients suffering from chronic pain exhibiting difficult behavior is likely much higher. Many of these patients suffer from depression and anxiety, and many have been victims of abuse. It is often clear to physicians or other providers immediately when they see these patients that they are difficult patients because of the feelings they elicit in the provider such as those described above.

These patients are often noncompliant and dissatisfied with treatment. They have idiosyncratic reactions to treatments. They often have somato-form disorders and may have issues with opioid misuse if not overt addiction. Difficult patients often have poor satisfaction with the care that providers give to them; they are often functionally limited and tend to use extraordinary amounts of health care resources. They can elicit feelings in their providers beyond frustration and dislike and can actually produces feeling of incompetency and anger in providers. It has been shown that the prevalence of cluster B personality disorders in chronic pain patients is higher than the incidence of personality disorders in prison parolees. They often have unrealistic expectations and believe that their pain should be eliminated. These patients are emotionally exhausting for providers and for all employees in the office or clinic. They can take up exorbitant amounts of time and cost providers money.

James Groves wrote of caring for "the hateful patient" in 1978 along with strategies that can be used to help manage them. Using Groves's difficult patient groups, the patient described above would be classified as an "entitled demander." Grove would suggest trying not to react to the patient's anger and to focus instead on trying to help the patient understand what realistic expectations are. If you can develop a doctor-patient relationship based on trust and confidence, then you may be able to succeed. Not all providers are skilled at handling difficult patients, but a commitment to trying to help a patient and a study of the subject can help improve those skills.

The physician above was willing to try to help the patient and scheduled regular appointments even though it was clear from the outset that the encounters were not going to be easy. If the provider had been able to sustain the relationship, he may have been able to, by empathic listening alone, prove that he appreciated that his patient was really suffering, and may have helped her develop more-realistic expectations, may have helped her to begin a course of exercise, and may have been able to convince her that multidisciplinary pain care involves specialists from a variety of disciplines including psychology and psychiatry.

The physician could have determined whether or not the patient was suffering from depression, anxiety, or had a different psychiatric problem, even borderline personality disorder, which may have responded to dialectical behavioral therapy. One of the important points here is that a committed provider could conceivably change his patient's life for the better despite the cost in time, effort, and provider emotion. The problem with difficult patients is as much about the patient's behaviors as it is about the provider's responses to them, and interest and ability to try to manage these patients. The provider described above may have worried about the patient. This patient's visits may have interrupted his sleep. The provider may have felt frustrated because he or she did not know how to manage the patient, and the provider felt guilty because he or she may have blamed himself for the poor relationship.

Success dealing with difficult patients really depends on the provider's ability to understand what precipitates the behaviors of their patients that give rise to the unpleasant feelings they evoke. Understanding chronic pain is crucial. Demonstrating empathy helps the patient feel heard and understood. Understanding comorbid psychopathology and their treatments, and understanding that it often requires a multidisciplinary team to help these patients can improve success.

KEY POINTS TO REMEMBER

- Caring for difficult patients requires skill, caring, patience, and a commitment to attempting to help someone who has been previously refractory to treatment.
- Psychopathology is common in patients suffering from chronic pain.

Further Reading

Wasan AD, Wootton J, Jamison RN. Dealing with difficult patients in your pain practice. *Reg Anesth Pain Med* 2005;30:184-192.

Treatment Overview

25 Antidepressants

A 45-year-old gentleman presents with a long-standing history of chronic pain including a diagnosis of complex regional pain syndrome, fibromyalgia, osteoarthritis of bilateral knees with continued moderate pain despite treatment with physical therapy, opioids, anticonvulsants, and procedural therapy. He continues to suffer from severe low back pain as well as myalgias and arthralgias in the upper and lower extremities that are not relieved with a standard medication regimen. His past medical history is significant for hypertension and oral medication controlled diabetes. Recently, he has lost the desire to participate in social activities with his friends, and his mood is depressed. He has been recently placed on amitriptyline, which caused a side effect of constipation, and he presents for further management of his painful condition as well as his depressed mood.

What do you do now?

The patient is suffering from chronic pain that has not responded to conservative treatment. The treatment has consisted of physical medicine, traditional analgesics including NSAIDs and opioids, as well as adjuvant analgesics including anticonvulsants, and recently antidepressants. His mood is quite affected by the complexity of his chronic pain condition, and as a result, his treatments should focus on functional rehabilitation, improvement in mood with psychological therapy including cognitive behavioral therapy, and antidepressants.

Antidepressants are adjuvant analgesics that are used for the treatment of pain, although their primary indications are for conditions other than pain. Adjuvant analgesics such as antidepressants are often coadministered with the traditional analgesics. There is a large body of evidence for the analgesic action of antidepressants in chronic, noncancer pain, but few data available for acute pain and cancer pain. The original reason for treatment of chronic pain with antidepressants appears to have been relief of concomitant depression. A portion of chronic pain patients have been noted to be depressed and have been shown to have an increased response to tricyclic antidepressants. Randomized control trials have demonstrated relief of both pain and depression with these agents.

Pain is transmitted from peripheral sites via A delta and C fibers, which in turn synapse in the dorsal horn of the spinal cord. Pain can be modulated by the activity of descending inhibitory fibers passing from the brain to the spinal cord. The neurotransmitters primarily involved in descending pathways (examples: norepinephrine and serotonin) are modulated by the antidepressants. Agents that block the reuptake of norepinephrine and serotonin at final dorsal horn synapses can lead to increased inhibition of pain. In addition to their central and peripheral nervous system effects for pain modulation, antidepressants can help to regulate sleep and control anxiety and depression, which may be contributing factors to the level of chronic pain. Imipramine is noted as the first antidepressant, which was discovered 40 years ago. There are more than 20 antidepressants on the market. Classic antidepressants include tricyclic antidepressants (TCAs), selective serotonin reuptake inhibitors (SSRIs), and mixed.

TRICYCLIC ANTIDEPRESSANTS (TCAS)

Tricyclic antidepressants' use for pain was first described by Lance and Curran, who did a placebo-controlled trial showing that amitriptyline reduced the severity of tension headaches. There are several studies that support efficacy of TCAs in treatment of postherpetic neuralgia, diabetic neuropathy, migraines, and other chronic pain conditions.

Adverse side effects with tricyclic antidepressants include:

- Cardiovascular side effects, such as postural hypotension, heart block, and arrhythmias.
- Anticholinergic and quinidine-like cardiac effects of TCAs cause serious reservations about their use in patients with preexisting conduction defects, cardiac ischemia, or myocardial infarction.
- Anticholinergic effects include dry mouth, urinary retention, and constipation. They have been associated with weight gain, sexual dysfunction, delirium, dissociated reactions, sedation, and aggravation of narrow-angle glaucoma.

There is more risk in the elderly or those on other anticholinergic drugs. Lowering TCA doses, discontinuing other drugs, or using a less-anticholinergic drug may be necessary in some patients. For patients starting on TCAs, an EKG is recommended (but not mandatory) prior to treatment.

SELECTIVE SEROTONIN REUPTAKE INHIBITORS (SSRIS)

SSRIs offer the advantages of greater tolerability of side effects and relative safety in overdoses compared with TCAs. The SSRIs may benefit some patients who fail to respond to TCAs, or who are at risk for side effects. Most SSRIs are free of anticholinergic, adrenergic, and histaminergic receptor actions. Thus, they are relatively unlikely to cause anticholinergic, autonomic, or cardiac side effects, as well as orthostatic hypotension, sedation, or weight gain. However, they do have side effects, which include insomnia, diarrhea, nausea, agitation, anxiety, exacerbations of mania or psychosis, sexual disturbances, headache, and tremor. Extrapyramidal side effects are rare, but have been reported with fluoxetine.

SSRI antidepressants are metabolized by and inhibit cytochrome 450 isoenzymes. Important interactions can occur with other psychotropic agents, antiarrhythmics, anticonvulsants, and anticoagulants.

SELECTIVE NOREPINEPHRINE REUPTAKE INHIBITORS (SNRIS)

SNRIs, such as venlafaxine and duloxetine, block reuptake of serotonin and norepinephrine, but are relatively free of muscurinic, anticholinergic, histaminic, and alpha adrenergic receptor effects. Venlafaxine lacks significant anticholinergic side effects and has been shown to be effective in the treatment of chronic pain. However, it has been associated with hypotension, exacerbating existing seizure disorders, and triggering mania. Duloxetine is the only antidepressant currently approved for neuropathic pain. Side effects include insomnia, nervousness, and anxiety. They have been associated with sedation, fatigue, headaches, nausea, vomiting, diarrhea, dyspepsia, sexual dysfunction, and hypoglycemia.

APPROACH TO THERAPY

For patients with chronic pain, starting on antidepressant therapy (see Table 25.1) in the midst of many failures from side effects, initial high dosing, noncompliance, or inadequate trials may be difficult. It is important to discuss with the patient goals of treatment and adverse effects while using antidepressants. Patients also need to be informed that starting doses will be low and slowly increased until satisfactory relief of pain or symptoms, or an intolerable adverse effect, is experienced. It is important to inform the patient that the effect of a dose increase may not be experienced for a week or so, and that side effects are probable, the most common being dry mouth, constipation, and drowsiness. Sedation may be useful in some patients with bedtime dosing, if insomnia is a problem.

It is important to note that a past medical history of glaucoma, prostate hypertrophy, and cardiovascular disease without arrhythmia should spark caution when using the antidepressant class. Useful baseline tests include blood pressure, liver and kidney function labs, electrolytes, hematology,

TABLE 25.1 **Antidepressants Used for Pain**

Medication	Starting Dose	Dose Range	Comments
		Tricyclic Antidepressants	
amitriptyline	25 mg po at bedtime 10 mg po for the elderly	10 to 150 mg po at bedtime	Side effects include dry mouth, drowsiness, dizziness, constipation, urinary retention, confusion. Titrate dose every few days to minimize side effects. *Caution* in the elderly and in patients with cardiovascular disease.
nortriptyline	25 mg po at bedtime 10 mg po for the elderly	10 to 150 mg po at bedtime	Lower side-effect profile than amitriptyline. Titrate as above.
desipramine	25 mg po at bedtime 10 mg po for the elderly	10 to 150 mg po at bedtime	
		Selective Serotonin Reuptake Inhibitors (SSRIs)	
fluoxetine	20 mg daily	20 to 80 mg daily	Should not use with MAO inhibitors. Consider lowering starting dose for patients for whom tolerability is a concern.
paroxetine	20 mg daily	20 to 60 mg daily	
sertraline	25 mg daily	25 to 200 mg daily	
		Selective Norepinephrine Reuptake Inhibitors (SNRIs)	
venlafaxine	25 mg daily	25 to 225 mg daily	Should not use with MAO inhibitors. Consider lowering starting dose for patients for whom tolerability is a concern.
duloxetine	20 mg daily	20 to 60 mg daily	

and EKG. Depending on patient's past medical history, an antidepressant should be selected based on the side-effect profile.

More comparative studies are needed to determine the relative efficacy of antidepressants and how they compare with other agents such as the anticonvulsants, opioids, and other treatment options; however, the antidepressants are often a part of the treatment for patients with chronic pain.

KEY POINTS TO REMEMBER

- Antidepressants are often part of the treatment for patients with chronic pain.
- When choosing an antidepressant, consider the patient's past medical history and the medication's side-effect profile.
- In the elderly, use caution when prescribing the TCAs, such as amitriptyline.

Further Reading

Atkinson JH Jr., Kremer EF, Risch SC, Janowsky DS. Basal and post-dexamethasone cortisol and prolactin concentrations in depressed and non-depressed patients with chronic pain syndromes. *Pain* 1986;25(1):23-34.

Couch JR, Ziegler DK, Hassanein R. Amitriptyline in the prophylaxis of migraine: effectiveness and relationship of antimigraine and antidepressant effects. *Neurology* 1976;26(2):121-127.

Glassman AH, Roose SP. Risks of antidepressants in the elderly: tricyclic antidepressants and arrhythmia-revising risks. *Gerontology* 1994;40(Suppl 1):15-20.

Lance JW, Curran DA. Treatment of chronic tension headache. *Lancet* 1964;1(7345): 1236-1239.

Lunn MP, Hughes RA, Wiffen PJ. Duloxetine for treating painful neuropathy or chronic pain. *Cochrane Database Syst Rev* 2009(4):CD007115.

Nemeroff CB, DeVane CL, Pollock BG. Newer antidepressants and the cytochrome P450 system. *Am J Psychiatry* 1996;153(3):311-320.

Okasha A, Ghaleb HA, Sadek A. A double blind trial for the clinical management of psychogenic headache. *Br J Psychiatry* 1973;122(567):181-183.

Roose SP, Glassman AH. Antidepressant choice in the patient with cardiac disease: lessons from the Cardiac Arrhythmia Suppression Trial (CAST) studies. *J Clin Psychiatry* 1994;55(Suppl A):83-87; discussion 88-89, 98-100.

Saarto T, Wiffen PJ. Antidepressants for neuropathic pain: a Cochrane review. *J Neurol Neurosurg Psychiatry* 2010;81(12):1372-1373.

Watson P, Chipman M, Monks R. *Antidepressant Analgesics: A Systematic Review and Comparative Study*, 5th ed. Elsevier Limited, China, 2006.

26 Anticonvulsants

A 21-year-old woman has severe neuropathic pain related to a lumbar herniated disc. She has a past medical history of Ehlers-Danlos syndrome, which is confounding her symptomatology. She describes pain in her lower extremity, predominantly on the right side. It radiates down the posterior aspect of her leg into her foot, and is described as severe, lancinating pain. Her pain is constant and unrelenting, requiring high-dose opioids for moderate pain control. She is currently taking oxycodone sustained release, amitriptyline, flexeril, and naproxen with only moderate pain relief. She had recently been trialed on gabapentin with increased doses causing sedation without decreasing her symptoms. She presents to the Pain Clinic for improvement in pain control.

What do you do now?

Anticonvulsant drugs, such as gabapentin, have been used in pain management long after they were introduced for the treatment of epilepsy. Both neuropathic pain and epilepsy are associated with changes in the sodium and calcium channel subunit expression resulting in functional changes. In chronic, neuropathic pain, the altered composition of sodium and calcium channels is thought to evoke firing at ectopic sites along the sensory pathway. The clinical impression, therefore, is that they are useful for neuropathic pain syndromes.

The precise mechanism of action and role by which anticonvulsant drugs function remains uncertain; however, there has been recent data that have offered various explanations. Anticonvulsants may modulate both peripheral and central components of pain by several routes including antagonism of sodium channels, inhibition of excitatory transmission as mediated by N-methyl-d-aspartate receptors, and enhancement of gamma-aminobutyric acid (GABA)-mediated inhibition.

Most of the clinically available anticonvulsants have the ability to block voltage-gated sodium channels in a use-dependent manner; however, there are other anticonvulsants that act on other ion channel systems. Anticonvulsant drugs show relatively wide ranges of values for number needed to treat (NNT) to produce analgesia (see Table 26.1; also see Table 26.2), and number needed to harm (NNH) to produce adverse effects.

ANTICONVULSANTS–PRIMARY MECHANISM OF ACTION INVOLVING VOLTAGE-GATED SODIUM CHANNELS

Carbamazepine

Carbamazepine is an oral anticonvulsant drug identified as a first-line treatment for trigeminal neuralgia. It is chemically related to the tricyclic antidepressants, as it inhibits noradrenaline uptake and modulates voltage-gated sodium channels.

Carbamazepine is metabolized in the liver. Adverse reactions include sedation, blurry vision, headaches, hepatitis, cholestasis, agranulocytosis, pancytopenia, aplastic anemia, rash, alopecia, Stevens-Johnson syndrome, oliguria, azotemia, and renal failure. Carbemazepine is used in the treatment of trigeminal neuralgia, diabetic neuropathy, and central pain.

TABLE 26.1 NNT (95% Confidence Interval) to Produce Analgesia

Disease State	Drug	NNT Values (95% Confidence Interval)
Trigeminal neuralgia	carbamazepine	2.5 (2.0-3.4)
Postherpetic neuralgia	gabapentin	3.2 (2.4-5.0)
Diabetic neuropathy	phenytoin	2.1 (1.5-3.6)
Diabetic neuropathy	carbamazepine	2.3 (1.6-3.8)
Diabetic neuropathy	gabapentin	3.8 (2.4-8.7)

Lamotrigine

Lamotrigine blocks voltage-dependent sodium channels and inhibits glutamate release from presynaptic neurons. It is an oral anticonvulsant drug that was approved by the FDA in 1994. Lamotrigine undergoes glucuronidation in the liver, and less than 10% of a dose is eliminated unchanged by the kidney. Dose adjustments are needed in patients with hepatic impairment. The most common adverse effect is rash, which can occur in up to 10% of patients, while 1 in 1,000 patients can develop Stevens-Johnson syndrome. Other side effects include dizziness, blurred vision, ataxia, nausea, and vomiting. Lamotrigine has shown some efficacy in treatment of trigeminal neuralgia, HIV neuropathy, diabetic neuropathy, central post-stroke pain, spinal cord injury, and mixed neuropathic pain.

Oxcarbazepine

Oxcarbazepine is a 10-keto analog of carbamazepine. Oxcarbazepine is completely absorbed and metabolized to its pharmacologically active metabolite, which is devoid of the toxicity seen with the metabolite of carbamazepine. Oxcarbazepine's mechanism of action includes binding to sodium channels in their inactive state, increasing potassium conductance, and modulating calcium channels. Comparison meta-analysis between oxcarbazepine and carbamazepine in trigeminal neuralgia was conducted by Beydoun in 2002. There were no significant differences in the two groups suffering from trigeminal neuralgia in global efficacy, weekly attacks, or evoked pain; however, tolerability was better with oxcarbazepine.

TABLE 26.2 **Anticonvulsants Used for Pain**

Medication	Starting Dose	Dose Range	Comments
Primary Mechanism of Action Involving Voltage-Gated Sodium Channels			
Carbamazepine	100 mg bid	200 to 1200mg/day in divided doses	Therapeutic plasma concentration between 8 to 12 mcg/ml
Lamotrigine	25 mg/day	100 mg/day	Dose adjustments are needed in patients with hepatic impairment. There are significant interactions with other anticonvulsants. Risk of Stevens-Johnson syndrome.
Oxcarbazepine	150 mg po bid	1200 mg po bid	Less toxicity as compared with carbamazepine
Topiramate	25 mg once daily	400mg/day in divided doses	Caution use in patient with history of nephrolithiasis.
Valproic acid	250 mg per day	2000 mg/day in divided doses	Routes of administration include intravenous and oral.
Anticonvulsants with Mechanism of Action Not Involving Voltage-Gated Sodium Channels			
Gabapentin	300 mg titrated to tid In the elderly, 100mg titrated to tid	3600 mg/day in divided doses	Dosage adjustments are necessary in patients with impaired renal function.
Pregabalin	25 titrated to tid	450 mg/day in divided doses	

Topiramate

Topiramate blocks voltage-gated sodium channels, augments GABA-mediated chloride current, blocks excitatory glutamate activity, increases potassium conductance, and inhibits carbonic anhdrase. Topiramate has a long duration of action in a narrow therapeutic window. It is not metabolized to a great extent; 70% of an administered dose is eliminated unchanged in the urine and therefore dose adjustments are needed in patients with chronic renal failure. The most commonly reported side effects are drowsiness, dizziness, ataxia, aphasia, and weight loss. Topiramate has the potential to interact with other drugs, reducing serum digoxin levels, and decreasing the efficacy of oral contraceptives. Phenytoin, carbamazepine, and barbiturates reduce topiramate serum concentrations.

A randomized, double-blind, placebo-controlled, multicenter trial with 323 patients evaluated topiramate in patients with painful diabetic neuropathy (Raskin et al., 2004). Topiramate was titrated to a tolerated dose over an 8-week period followed by a 4-week maintenance period, and it resulted in statistically significant lower pain scores at the final visit compared with scores from those who received placebo.

Valproic Acid

Valproic acid blocks sodium channels and augments GABA(A). It is commonly used in the treatment of migraine, cluster, and tension headaches, however, there are conflicting reports on its efficacy with neuropathic pain. Valproic acid's side effects include GI upset, CNS effects, hematologic toxicity, rashes, alterations in liver function tests, and weight gain. It requires frequent monitoring during the first year, and can be associated with spina bifida in fetuses of patients who are pregnant. Valproic acid is rapidly absorbed with a peak serum level within 1 to 4 hours, and a half-life of 10 hours. It is highly bound to albumin, and is excreted in the urine.

ANTICONVULSANTS WITH MECHANISM OF ACTION NOT INVOLVING VOLTAGE-GATED SODIUM CHANNELS

Gabapentin

Gabapentin was introduced in the United States in 1994 as an anticonvulsant. It is a structural analog of GABA(A) but it does not modify GABA, instead it binds to calcium channels. It is not actively metabolized, but rather eliminated from the systemic circulation by renal excretion as an unchanged drug. The elimination half-life is 5 to 7 hours, and renal clearance is directly proportional to creatinine clearance. Dosage adjustments are necessary in patients with impaired renal function; however, it can be removed by hemodialysis. The most common side effects are sedation, dizziness, somnolence, nausea, vomiting, and edema.

Multicenter, randomized, placebo-controlled studies have shown efficacy of gabapentin in treatment of postherpetic neuralgia, diabetic neuropathy, refractory or complex regional pain syndrome Type I, and migraine headaches. It has been found effective in reducing the pain associated with multiple sclerosis. In addition, it appeared to improve the analgesic effects of opioids in patients with neuropathic cancer pain. The FDA has approved gabapentin for the treatment of postherpetic neuralgia.

Pregabalin

Pregabalin is a GABA analog, and like gabapentin, it binds to calcium channels. Pregabalin has an improved pharmacokinetic profile over gabapentin. Side effects include dizziness, drowsiness, blurred vision, dry mouth, edema, and weight gain.

Double-blind studies have shown pregabalin to be effective in the management of painful diabetic neuropathy as well as postherpetic neuralgia.

KEY POINTS TO REMEMBER

- Anticonvulsants have shown efficacy for analgesia and are often part of the treatment for patients with chronic pain.
- Lamotrigine can cause a side effect of rash and in rare cases, Stevens-Johnson syndrome.
- Topiramate should be used with caution in patients with a history of nephrolithiasis secondary to its carbonic anhydrase inhibition.
- When choosing an anticonvulsant, consider the patient's past medical history and the medication's side-effect profile.
- Gabapentin has been FDA approved for the treatment of postherpetic neuralgia.

Further Reading

Backonja M, Glanzman RL. Gabapentin dosing for neuropathic pain: evidence from randomized, placebo-controlled clinical trials. *Clin Ther* 2003;25(1):81-104.

Beydoun A, Kutluay E. Oxcarbazepine. *Expert Opin Pharmacother* 2002;3(1):59-71.

Dworkin RH, Corbin AE, Young JP Jr., et al. Pregabalin for the treatment of postherpetic neuralgia: a randomized, placebo-controlled trial. *Neurology* 2003;60(8):1274-1283.

Eisenberg E, Lurie Y, Braker C, Daoud D, Ishay A. Lamotrigine reduces painful diabetic neuropathy: a randomized, controlled study. *Neurology* 2001;57(3):505-509.

Gorson KC, Schott C, Herman R, Ropper AH, Rand WM. Gabapentin in the treatment of painful diabetic neuropathy: a placebo controlled, double blind, crossover trial. *J Neurol Neurosurg Psychiatry* 1999;66(2):251-252.

Mao J, Chen LL. Gabapentin in pain management. *Anesth Analg* 2000;91(3):680-687.

Raskin P, Donofrio PD, Rosenthal NR, et al. Topiramate vs placebo in painful diabetic neuropathy: analgesic and metabolic effects. *Neurology* 2004;63(5):865-873.

Richter RW, Portenoy R, Sharma U, Lamoreaux L, Bockbrader H, Knapp LE. Relief of painful diabetic peripheral neuropathy with pregabalin: a randomized, placebo-controlled trial. *J Pain* 2005;6(4):253-260.

Sabatowski R, Galvez R, Cherry DA, et al. Pregabalin reduces pain and improves sleep and mood disturbances in patients with post-herpetic neuralgia: results of a randomised, placebo-controlled clinical trial. *Pain* 2004;109(1-2):26-35.

Sang C, Hayes K. *Anticonvulsant Medications in Neuropathic Pain*, 5th ed. Elsevier Limited, China, 2006.

White HS. Comparative anticonvulsant and mechanistic profile of the established and newer antiepileptic drugs. *Epilepsia* 1999;40 (Suppl 5):S2-10.

Wiffen P, Collins S, McQuay H, Carroll D, Jadad A, Moore A. Anticonvulsant drugs for acute and chronic pain. *Cochrane Database Syst Rev* 2005(3):CD001133.

Wiffen PJ, McQuay HJ, Edwards JE, Moore RA. Gabapentin for acute and chronic pain. *Cochrane Database Syst Rev* 2005(3):CD005452.

27 Opioids

A 32-year-old woman presents with a 3-month history of pain behind her right ear. There was no antecedent injury or event. She developed right facial paralysis, tingling in her face, a "wave" noise in her right ear, and decreased sensation on the side of her tongue. As her pain intensifies, she develops lacrimation in her right eye. She denies having had a rash. She has a gold weight implanted in her right eye lid.

She was initially treated with prednisone, current dose of 80 mg per day, however, when she attempts to decrease her dose, her pain dramatically increases. In addition, she is using amitriptyline 100 mg at bedtime and had been using gabapentin, but it was discontinued secondary to new onset tachycardia and sedation, which did gradually diminish after the taper. However, despite her medication change, she continues to complain of dry mouth, orthostatic hypotension, episodic tachycardia, and exhaustion.

She has a past medical history of hypertension, which has been elevated since starting prednisone; her blood pressure during her office visit is 149/100. She was working full time as an RN but had to stop because of her recent difficulty with sleep, exhaustion, and anxiety.

She has been diagnosed with a highly vascular acoustic neuroma. The tumor was so vascular that her surgeons wanted to wait six months to repeat her MRI before deciding on a surgical plan.

She presents to clinic for pain management while awaiting a surgical plan.

What do you do now?

This patient is suffering from neuropathic pain related to tumor involvement with at least one cranial nerve. The mainstay of treatment from a pharmacological perspective for neuropathic pain is a combination of anticonvulsants, antidepressants, and opioid analgesics. She is suffering from dramatic side effects from her current regiment, specifically orthostatic hypotension, intermittent tachycardia, and dry mouth from the amitriptyline; and anxiety, sleeplessness, and elevated blood pressure from the prednisone. Both of these drugs should be weaned and a trial of drugs initiated with similar efficacy but fewer side effects.

The patient was initially advised to wean off of the amitriptyline over the course of 2 weeks and she was given a prescription for duloxetine 30 mg daily and pregabalin 50 mg three times a day. In addition, she was started on an opioid, methadone at 2.5 mg every 8 hours.

There is currently indisputable evidence supporting the use opioids for the treatment of neuropathic pain despite the fact that there may have been controversy over this practice a decade ago. In addition, there is excellent evidence supporting the use of many anticonvulsants and antidepressants, both noradrenergic and serotonergic reuptake inhibitors.

OPIOIDS AND NEUROPATHIC PAIN

At the time of diagnosis, despite the high dose of steroids, her Brief Pain Inventory (BPI) severity score was 5.3 on 0 to 10 scale and her BPI interference score was 7.3 on a 0 to 10 scale. The BPI is a validated and reliable instrument that takes into account worst pain, least pain, average pain, and a variety of other indices and translates it into a single number "Severity Score" on a 0 to 10 scale. Similarly the BPI interference scale is a measure of how much pain interferes with various elements of function.

As stated previously, methadone was selected as the opioid analgesic because theoretically it may be efficacious for the treatment of neuropathic pain due to its NMDA receptor antagonist properties. Other advantages of methadone relative to other opioids are its cost, which is approximately 1/10 as much as a comparable dose of any other opioid. Methadone is a relatively long acting opioid, the analgesic duration of action of methadone is between 6 and 8 hours. Its elimination half-life is quite long, in the 48-hour range, and this discrepancy is due to the fact that methadone is highly liquid soluble.

In addition, it has both an alpha and beta elimination half-life, the alpha half-life being related to redistribution into fatty tissue accounting for the short analgesic duration of action and the beta elimination half-life related to accumulation of the drug in fatty and other tissue. This long beta elimination half-life accounts for the need to be knowledgeable and cautious about the use of methadone. If doses are increased more often than approximately every 10 days there can be "stacking" of doses. This means that the dose may be increased when a steady state serum level has not yet been reached, which could result in an overdose. A reasonable starting dose for a young opioid naive patient is 2.5 mg three times per day. If this patient were over the age of 60, a starting dose might be 2.5 mg once a day.

This patient was instructed to increase her duloxetine dose to a target dose of 60 mg per day and her pregabalin to a target dose of 150 mg three times per day. Her methadone was gradually increased over the course of 2 months to 15 mg three times per day. Her BPI pain and interference scores were both 2 on a 0 to 10 scale within approximately 1 month of the time of initiation of these treatments. Her prednisone dose was gradually weaned off over approximately 6 months. The patient's pain scores increased slightly during this period of time but were always much lower than the initial pain scores. Her blood pressure stabilized at 120/74.

OPIOID SIDE EFFECTS

The most worrisome side effect of opioid therapy is addiction. Some studies have shown that up to 50% of patients seen in pain centers in the United States have urine toxicology results inconsistent with reported use of drug and/or demonstrates signs or symptoms consistent with addiction. Diversion is an important issue, and there are estimates that up to 25% of opioids prescribed by physicians are diverted. Abuse can occur in the absence of addiction. An example of abuse might be taking an increased dose of opioid periodically for its euphoric effect but without really meeting DSM-IV criteria for a diagnosis of addiction. Misuse occurs when patients take a dose of opioids to help them sleep or in a nonprescribed fashion, for example, increasing the dose because the prescribed dose does not control the pain immediately. It is extremely important to have a discussion about addiction and all of the other side effects of opioid use with patients prior to prescribing to them to ensure their safety and to document that discussion either in the form of an opioid agreement or a comprehensive note.

Constipation is an extremely important side effect that needs to be managed with patients treated with opioids. A conversation about constipation and a plan for management should be discussed at the time of the initiation of opioid therapy. Prune juice, bran cereal, and senna teas are readily available and in most cases will maintain effective bowel motility, but often laxatives are required, particularly in elderly patients.

Other potential side effects include sedation, sexual dysfunction, osteoporosis, and fracture.

OPIOID PRESCRIPTION MONITORING

Assessment is an essential part of determining who might be a candidate for long-term opioid therapy. This patient was a low risk candidate based on the following:

- She had no prior history of alcoholism or drug abuse.
- She had a negative family history for alcoholism or drug abuse.
- She was working full-time.
- She did not smoke cigarettes.
- She had objective evidence of a painful disorder.

A difference in any one of the above items would have placed her at moderate or high risk for developing a problem with addiction, diversion, abuse, or misuse. The patient at moderate risk, for example, a patient's whose only risk factor is cigarette smoking or a family history of alcoholism or patients at high risk, for example, a patient with a personal history of alcoholism or drug abuse can still be treated with opioids, but it requires special attention and effort. There should be an increased educational component to care of moderate and high risk patients.

Monitoring patients treated with opioids for compliance and side effects is equally important as assessment. Urine toxicology testing is an essential component of their care, and in fact a patient at high risk should probably have a urine toxicology specimen tested on a monthly basis. Patients at high risk may need to be seen more frequently, even more than once a month and be given prescriptions for smaller aliquots of drugs. It is also important to remember that any patient who is treated with opioids is treated on a trial basis and there needs to be clear, explicitly enunciated goals of treatment, and if those goals are not met then patients should be weaned off of opioids.

Decision making should always be individualized but, as a general rule of thumb, a patient who does not have objective evidence of a painful disorder and is high risk should probably not be treated with opioids.

KEY POINTS TO REMEMBER

- Neuropathic pain usually responds to a combination of anticonvulsants, antidepressants, and opioids.
- Opioids can usually be used effectively and safely but require individualization of drug and dose, a skilled assessment of risk and risk stratification, and continual monitoring for side effects.
- Reliable and validated survey instruments are available to gauge the effectiveness of treatment.
- High risk patients without objective evidence of a painful disorder should probably not be treated with opioids.

Further Reading

Chou R, Fanciullo GJ, Fine PG, et al. Opioid treatment guidelines: clinical guidelines for the use of chronic opioid therapy in chronic noncancer pain. *J Pain* 2009;10(2):113-130.

Katz N, Sherburne S, Vielguth J, Rose RJ, Fanciullo GJ. Behavioral monitoring and urine toxicology testing in patients receiving long-term opioid therapy. *Anesth Analg* 2003;97:1097-1102.

Keller S, Bann CM, Dodd SL, Schein J, Mendoza TR, Cleeland CS. Validity of the Brief Pain Inventory for use in documenting the outcomes of patients with noncancer pain. *Clin J Pain* 2004;20(5):309-318.

28 Other Adjuvant Drugs

A 60-year-old male with a history of a right knee injury resulting in osteoarthritis and subsequent right total knee replacement continues to suffer from right knee pain. His pain has been refractory to physical therapy, opioids including morphine sustained release, and gabapentin. His past medical history is significant for hypertension and depression. His mood has been affected by his chronic pain issues, and he was recently placed on duloxetine with minimal benefit. He continues to suffer from right knee pain, which he describes as aching, throbbing pain, with occasional severe spasms in his calves. He presents to his primary care physician's office for further treatment options regarding his pain.

What do you do now?

The patient has significant pain that has not responded to conservative treatment with opioids, physical therapy, anticonvulsants, and antidepressants. At this time, there is no mention of other adjuvant analgesics for his pain symptoms, and therefore the treating provider should address and treat as necessary.

The traditional analgesics are nonopioids (for example, NSAIDs) and opioids. Adjuvant analgesics are drugs in which the primary indications are for conditions other than pain, but are being used in the management of chronic pain. In some clinical settings, such as in patients with postherpetic neuralgia, trigeminal neuralgia, and painful polyneuropathies, they are accepted as a first-line drug. In the *analgesic ladder*, best pain relief may be obtained if all components of the ladder are used simultaneously, in the sense that one analgesic for one drug class adds to the analgesia provided by another drug class. Adjuvant analgesics include antidepressants (discussed in chapter 25), anticonvulsants (discussed in chapter 26), local anesthetics, alpha-2 adrenergic agonists, *N*-methyl-d-aspartate (NMDA) receptor antagonists, and topical agents. Including these medications in an analgesic regimen may prove to be beneficial for pain control.

LOCAL ANESTHETICS

Local anesthetics (LA) in the form of IV, oral, or topical agents (creams, gels, patches), have been used for years for treatment of various chronic pain conditions. These include lidocaine, bupivacaine, and mexiletine.

LAs belong to the anti-arrhythmic group of medications and are used to treat arrhythmias of the heart, but have been used in patients experiencing refractory pain. They adhere to peripheral nerves and reduce pain signals carried from the peripheral nervous system to the central nervous system and brain. Mexiletine, in particular, has efficacy in the treatment of muscle stiffness disorders such as myotonia congenita or myotonic dystrophies. Mexiletine is used experimentally to treat pain associated with different kinds of peripheral neuropathy and has not been FDA approved.

ALPHA-2 ADRENERGIC AGONISTS

Alpha-2 adrenoreceptors (A2A) are located in primary afferent terminals, neurons in the superficial lamina of the spinal cord, and within several brainstem nuclei. Tizanadine and clonidine have utility as a pain reliever.

Clonidine produces analgesia at alpha adrenoreceptors in the spinal cord; it blocks conduction of C and A delta pain fibers, increases potassium conductance, and intensifies conduction blockade of local anesthetic. It is possible to achieve analgesia from systemic, epidural, or intrathecal administration of clonidine. Side effects include hypotension secondary to reduced sympathetic drive, bradycardia, and sedation. Clonidine has been used to treat neuropathic pain that is not responding to other treatment or therapy.

Tizanidine has been FDA approved as a muscle relaxant. It is used to treat spasms, cramping, and tightness of muscle caused by various conditions including multiple sclerosis, spasticity, back pain, or other injuries to the central nervous system. Side effects include hypotension and liver damage, therefore, patients treated with this drug should have baseline and regular liver function tests (LFTs) within the first six months of treatment. Tizanidine can cause sedation and has a potential to interact with other CNS depressants.

NMDA RECEPTOR ANTAGONISTS

NMDA is one of the newly discovered modulators in the spinal cord. The NMDA receptors function to cause changes in the hyperexcitability of the dorsal horn neuron, resulting in allodynia and hyperalgesia. Allodynia is pain produced by a non-noxious stimulus, and hyperalgesia is exacerbated pain produced by a noxious stimuli. NMDA receptor antagonists are useful in reducing opiate tolerance and hyperalgesia related to various painful conditions.

Ketamine is an anesthetic agent that blocks NMDA receptors and inhibits allodynia and hyperalgesia. Ketamine can be given by multiple routes including IV, IM, subcutaneous, oral, and transdermal. Orally administered ketamine undergoes extensive first-pass metabolism. Low-dose ketamine is recommended for its potential effectiveness in the treatment of complex regional pain syndrome according to a retrospective review published in *Pain Medicine* in 2004. Although low-dose ketamine therapy is established as a generally safe procedure, there are side effects in some patients which included hallucinations, dizziness, lightheadedness, and nausea.

Dextromethorphan is an oral antitussive that blocks NMDA receptors. It is associated with serotonin syndrome symptoms, which can include confusion, excitement, nervousness, restlessness, irritability, nausea, vomiting, and dysarthria. Dextromethorphan is also being studied as a possible treatment for neuropathic and fibromyalgia associated pain. It should be used with caution in patients taking monoamine oxidase inhibitors (MAOIs) or serotonin reuptake inhibitors due to the potential for serotonin syndrome, which is a potentially life-threatening condition that can occur rapidly due to a buildup of excessive amounts of serotonin in the body.

TOPICAL AGENTS

Topical agents can be used at the site of pain to alleviate symptoms. There have been multiple agents that have been used and compounded for treatment, for example, lidocaine, prilocaine, capsaicin, nonsteroidal anti-inflammatories, doxepin, amitriptyline, baclofen, gabapentin, ketamine, methyl salicylate (which can increase coumadin effects), and others.

A 5% lidocaine patch has been used for pain reduction in patients with postherpetic neuralgia. It is prescribed as 12 hours on and 12 hours off with a maximum of three patches at a time secondary to its toxicity. The patch can be cut to fit in a well-circumscribed area.

Capsaicin causes sensory nerve C-fibers to deplete their substance P. It is available as a topical cream (0.025% or 0.075%) which can be used 4 to 5 times daily. Most patients begin to see results within a few weeks of treatment. Its limited usefulness occurs secondary to initial burning upon application and subsequent intolerance by the patients. The frequency, treatments, and the painful side effect limit the compliance of this particular medication.

CONCLUSION

Adjuvant agents have been used for years for pain control in patients with acute, subacute, and chronic pain who are not responding to traditional analgesics such as NSAIDs or opioids.

- Adjuvant agents have shown efficacy for analgesia and are often part of the treatment for patients with chronic pain.
- Tizanadine can cause liver dysfunction, therefore LFTs should be monitored.
- Dextromethorphan should be used with caution in patients taking monoamine oxidase inhibitors (MAOIs) or serotonin reuptake inhibitors, due to the potential for serotonin syndrome.
- When choosing an adjuvant drug, consider the patient's past medical history and the medication's side-effect profile.

Further Reading

Cottingham R, Thomson K. Use of ketamine in prolonged entrapment. *J Accid Emerg Med* 1994;11(3):189–191.

Moore RA, Tramer MR, Carroll D, Wiffen PJ, McQuay HJ. Quantitative systematic review of topically applied non-steroidal anti-inflammatory drugs. *BMJ* 1998;316(7128): 333–338.

Robbins WR, Staats PS, Levine J, et al. Treatment of intractable pain with topical large-dose capsaicin: preliminary report. *Anesth Analg* 1998;86(3):579–583.

29 Spinal Cord Stimulation and Peripheral Nerve Stimulation

A 41-year-old woman with a history of L4 through S1 spinal fusion for low back pain and lumbar radiculopathy develops a reoccurrence of her symptoms 2 years post-op. She has been treated conservatively with anticonvulsants, antidepressants, opioids, and procedural therapy without benefit. A recent MRI shows no further operable cause of her pain. She is referred to the pain clinic for evaluation for spinal cord stimulation.

What do you do now?

The patient has failed multiple treatments including anticonvulsants, antidepressants, opioids, physical medicine, and interventional treatment. An MRI has ruled out additional surgical needs regarding her lumbar spine, but she continues to suffer from severe intractable pain. The strategy for this patient is spinal cord stimulation to control her back and lower extremity pain. Spinal cord stimulation, as well as peripheral nerve stimulation, can be an efficacious, cost effective option that can be used within the treatment continuum in many disease states.

Spinal cord stimulation (SCS) has been used since the 1960s to treat pain, with the first implantation for chronic cancer pain. As a result of advancements in technology, SCS as well as peripheral nerve stimulation (PNS) have been used for pain relief. A 20-year literature review found evidence for long-term safety and efficacy in various chronic pain conditions.

SPINAL CORD STIMULATION

Indications

There are various disease processes and painful conditions for which spinal cord stimulation has been shown to be effective, including chronic radicular pain, complex regional pain syndrome Types I and II, painful peripheral neuropathies, arachnoiditis, failed back surgery syndrome (FBSS), postherpetic neuralgia, painful peripheral vascular disease not amenable to surgery, and refractory angina pectoris. In addition, there are disease processes that have low probability of successful pain reduction including neuropathic pain following spinal cord injury, central pain (for example post-stroke pain, see chapter 4), avulsion injuries (for example brachial plexus avulsion, see chapter 7), axial low back pain, and phantom limb pain (see chapter 12).

The decision to implant a spinal cord stimulator (SCS) is based on selection criteria. It is used in the continuum of a patient's chronic intractable pain where other modalities have failed. Prior to implantation, patients are subjected to a physical and psychological evaluation, and diagnosis and imaging review by a multidisciplinary team. In addition, patients are screened for bleeding disorders, active systemic infections, infections at the site of the implant, untreated drug addiction issues, and psychological stability.

Trial and Implantation

The patient should have a successful trial of stimulation resulting in reduction of pain and improvement in function. The trial is performed with one to three epidural percutaneous leads or with a surgical paddle lead, and placed in the target zone based on the patients symptoms (see Figure 29.1). The trial period can range from hours to days depending on patient response and physician preference.

If the patient meets the criteria and has a successful trial, then the leads and generator will be implanted. By using a percutaneous or surgical approach, the SCS leads are placed within the epidural space of the lumbar, thoracic, or cervical spine depending on the patient's symptoms. Subsequently, the leads are tunneled under the skin and attached to an implantable programmable generator (IPG) in the subcutaneous tissue in the buttock area or at times in the lumbar musculature or chest. The IPG and the leads are connected and both incisional sites are closed.

The most common adverse events include lead migration, infection, swelling and redness, device failure leading to revisions, CSF leakage,

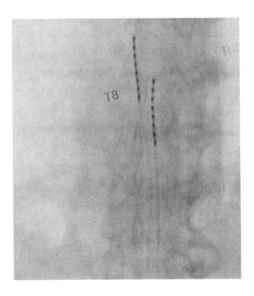

FIGURE 29.1 Radiographic imaging of patient with bilateral percutaneous leads placed in the thoracic region for lower extremity symptoms. (Courtesy of Tabitha A. Washington, MD, MS, Department of Anesthesiology, Section of Pain Medicine, Dartmouth Hitchcock Medical Center, Lebanon, NH.)

and/or hematoma. In addition, once a patient is implanted MRIs are contraindicated, therefore, prior to implantation the risk of future MRIs needs to be discussed.

Principals of Neurostimulation

Implantation of SCS devices involves placement of electrodes in target areas, thereby providing antidromic (normal direction) stimulation of the large fibers in the dorsal column (also referred to as dorsal column stimulator, or DCS). This may activate the proposed gating mechanism in the dorsal horn of the spinal cord, which causes suppression of acute and chronic pain. In ischemic extremity pain, the SCS may act to decrease ischemia by increasing or redistributing blood flow to the ischemic area or by decreasing tissue oxygen demand. Other hypothesized theories for the mechanism of SCS include reducing sympathetic outflow in patients with complex regional pain syndrome and improving organ function by stimulating intrinsic cardiac neurons in angina pectoris.

Conclusion

Spinal cord stimulation is a reversible and minimally invasive approach to treating chronic pain with the goals of reducing suffering, improving function, reducing healthcare utilization, and improving quality of life. They have been shown to be efficacious and cost effective in comparative therapies and are often considered a viable option for the treatment of various chronic pain conditions.

PERIPHERAL NERVE STIMULATION

Indications

Peripheral nerve stimulation is a neuromodulation technique in which an electrical current is applied to the peripheral nerves to reduce chronic pain conditions. It was first described in the 1960s, and a variety of techniques have been developed since that time.

Peripheral nerve stimulation (PNS) is indicated for the treatment of chronic pain localized to a peripheral nerve distribution that is not amendable to conservative treatment. It is useful for treating pain that is not accessible by spinal cord stimulation. It has efficacy for common disorders such as trigeminal, occipital, supraorbital, and inguinal neuralgia.

The overall strategy is similar to other forms of neurostimulation (see above, "Spinal Cord Stimulation" section).

Trial and Implantation

The trial period includes percutaneous or surgical placement of electrodes as indicated. If sufficient pain relief occurs, then a permanent system is implanted. Percutaneous or surgical paddle leads are used; however, surgical paddle leads seem to be less prone to migration, as the electrodes may be located in areas of excessive movement. In occipital and trigeminal neuralgia, individual leads are placed under the skin overlying the nerves, and intraoperative testing confirms the stimulation and parenthesia is in the appropriate location. For larger peripheral nerves, which are often deeper, an open approach is generally used (see Figure 29.2). Permanent leads are connected to an implantable pulse generator (see Figures 29.3 and 29.4).

Outcome

High quality published studies reporting the results of PNS are not abundant; however, it has successfully been used in the treatment of chronic pain. One review of published literature concerning occipital nerve stimulation reported the results of over 300 occipital nerve stimulators being used to treat headaches of various types with close to a 70% success rate.

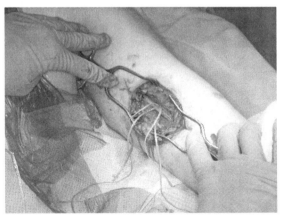

FIGURE 29.2 Open surgical approach for identifying the median and radial nerves for lead placement in a patient with neuralgia. (Courtesy of Gilbert J. Fanciullo, MD, MS, Department of Anesthesiology, Section of Pain Medicine, Dartmouth Hitchcock Medical Center, Lebanon, NH.)

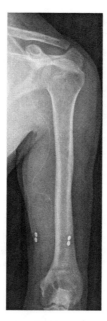

FIGURE 29.3 Radiographic imaging of patient with leads placed on the median and radial nerves in a patient with neuralgia. (Courtesy of Ralph Beasley, MD, Department of Anesthesiology, Section of Pain Medicine, Dartmouth Hitchcock Medical Center, Lebanon, NH.)

Conclusion

Peripheral nerve stimulation has a growing body of evidence and clinical data that suggests that it is a good approach to providing improvement in a patient's quality of life and function and for reducing suffering in patients with peripheral disease not amendable to conservative treatment.

KEY POINTS TO REMEMBER

- Spinal cord and peripheral nerve stimulation are used in the continuum of a patient's chronic intractable pain where other modalities have failed.
- SCS involves an electrical current applied to the dorsal column of the spinal cord from leads placed within the epidural space.
- PNS involves an electrical current applied to the peripheral nerves.
- MRIs are contraindicated once a SCS or PNS is implanted.

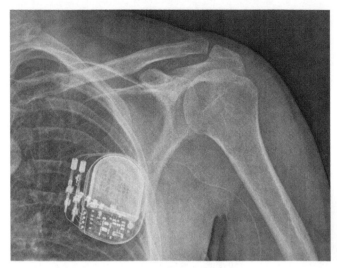

FIGURE 29.4 Radiographic imaging of patient with implantable pulse generator placed in the chest in a patient with neuralgia. (Courtesy of Ralph Beasley, MD, Department of Anesthesiology, Section of Pain Medicine, Dartmouth Hitchcock Medical Center, Lebanon, NH.)

Further Reading

Augustinsson LE, Carlsson CA, Holm J, Jivegard L. Epidural electrical stimulation in severe limb ischemia. Pain relief, increased blood flow, and a possible limb-saving effect. *Ann Surg* 1985;202(1):104-110.

Cameron T. Safety and efficacy of spinal cord stimulation for the treatment of chronic pain: a 20-year literature review. *J Neurosurg* 2004;100(3 Suppl Spine):254-267.

Foreman RD, Linderoth B, Ardell JL, et al. Modulation of intrinsic cardiac neurons by spinal cord stimulation: implications for its therapeutic use in angina pectoris. *Cardiovasc Res* 2000;47(2):367-375.

Jasper JF, Hayek SM. Implanted occipital nerve stimulators. *Pain Physician* 2008; 11(2):187-200.

Kumar K, Taylor RS, Jacques L, et al. Spinal cord stimulation versus conventional medical management for neuropathic pain: a multicentre randomised controlled trial in patients with failed back surgery syndrome. *Pain* 2007;132(1-2):179-188.

Levy R, Deer TR, Henderson J. Intracranial neurostimulation for pain control: a review. *Pain Physician* 2010;13(2):157-165.

Linderoth B, Meyerson B. Peripheral and central nervous system stimulation in chronic therapy-resistant pain. Background, hypothetical mechanisms and clinical experiences [in Swedish]. *Lakartidningen* 2001;98(47):5328-5334, 5336.

Quigley DG, Arnold J, Eldridge PR, et al. Long-term outcome of spinal cord stimulation and hardware complications. *Stereotact Funct Neurosurg* 2003;81(1-4):50-56.

Shealy CN, Mortimer JT, Reswick JB. Electrical inhibition of pain by stimulation of the dorsal columns: preliminary clinical report. *Anesth Analg* 1967;46(4):489-491.

30 Neurosurgical Procedures for Pain

A 23-year-old male with a past medical history of a fall off a 4-story building roof presents to the pain clinic with persistent shooting pain in his right leg 3 years following a L4 laminectomy and discectomy for similar pain. The patient has been trialed on anticonvulsants, antidepressants, and narcotic therapy without significant symptom or functional improvement. He is on disability but would like to return to work if possible. In spite of prolonged therapy in a functional restoration program, he continues to have debilitating radiculopathic pain. Repeat MRI of the lumbar spine shows no change from his previous MRI following his surgery. The patient was trialed with a 2 lead spinal cord stimulator and had good coverage for his right leg radicular pain. A permanent device was implanted, and the patient now feels much improved.

What do you do now?

Neurosurgical techniques have long been used for the treatment of intractable pain. They have been considered the most logical treatment choice for pain in that they would block pain pathways and thus prevent the transmission of pain signals to the cortex. However, as we have learned over time, the processing of pain is much more complex and includes not only stimulation of the pain pathways, but also the perception and psychological management of pain.

Over time, neurosurgical techniques have become more sophisticated and there are now multiple modalities being used to treat similar pain states. Because of this, there is difficulty finding consensus about which neurosurgical technique would best fit the treatment of certain pain states and if used, how to best measure "success" in a standardized fashion.

INDICATIONS

Intractable pain is pain that persists after all other therapies, other than neurosurgery, have been utilized and have not provided adequate relief of pain for a time period of at least 6 months; although, some use a duration of greater than 1 or 2 years.

The quality of pain may be characterized as either neuropathic or nociceptive:

- **Neuropathic pain** can be central or peripheral in origin; associated with allodynia, and is often described as lancinating, burning, or tingling. Some examples of neuropathic pain include: thalamic pain; post-stroke pain; phantom limb pain; pain due to multiple sclerosis, Parkinson's disease, syringomyelia, brachial plexus avulsion, and entrapment neuropathies; and spinal cord injury pain.
- **Nociceptive pain** is pain that is caused by tissue damage that gives rise to somatic or visceral stimuli. Often, this type of pain is well localized and characterized as aching, sharp, or cramping. This type of pain, in general, is responsive to NSAIDs, steroids, and analgesics.

Choosing the right patient for a neurosurgical technique is critical. There are multiple issues to consider before scheduling, including:

- Pain duration and nature of symptoms.
- Psychological stability of the patient.

- Patient expectation, including whether the patient is willing to accept that the procedure trial may be a failure.
- Patient's understanding of procedure risk, including device failure and infection that may result in removal of the hardware
- Discussion with patient regarding need for future imaging studies, as MRI requirements may preclude hardware placement.

Neurosurgical techniques for the treatment of pain can be classified into one of two categories: ablative or non-ablative (Table 30.1). However, ablative techniques have their disadvantages, they are irreversible, and have shown that over time (months to several years) there may be loss of the initial analgesic effect.

ABLATIVE TECHNIQUES

Peripheral Neurectomy

This technique involves the partial or complete resection of a cranial or peripheral nerve. From a technical standpoint, they are simple to perform, however complications can include motor weakness, anesthesia, loss of proprioception

TABLE 30.1 **Classifications of Surgical Techniques**

Ablative techniques injure or partially destroy the nerve

- Thermocoagulation; the process of applying radiofrequency or constant current through the tip of a nonpermanent electrode to damage peripheral nerves.
- Cryoprobe ablation.
- Alcohol and formalin injections.
- Peripheral neurectomy.
- Dorsal root ganglionectomy
- Dorsal root entry zone (DREZ) lesions.
- Sympathectomy.
- Midline myelotomy.
- Cordotomy.
- Intracranial ablations.
- Cingulotomy.

Non-ablative techniques spare the function of the nerve

- Decompression procedures.
- Spinal Cord and Peripheral Nerve Stimulators (see chapter 29).

and development of decubiti and Charcot joints. Deafferentation and neuropathic pain can also develop, as well as neuromas, which may require decompression. Months to years after the initial lesion, sprouting of adjacent sensory nerves restores sensation.

Dorsal Root Ganglionectomy

Initially used for intractable radicular pain and most recently for severe sciatica; dorsal root ganglionectomy involves the resection of the dorsal root ganglion. Side effects include bladder and bowel dysfunction that may require colostomy and/or urinary diversion, recurrence of pain over months to years, and deafferentation pain in up to 60% of patients. This deafferentation pain is most often amenable to treatment with oral analgesics and appears to be self-limited in most cases. It has also been shown to have limited efficacy in the treatment of noncancer pain such as C2 ganglionectomy for headache. For the treatment of cancer pain, there has been a 50–90% success rate, especially for the relief of pain associated with pelvic cancer, chest wall invasion, or multilevel ganglionectomy for brachial plexus invasion.

Dorsal Root Entry Zone (DREZ) Lesions

DREZ lesions were originally performed for treatment of chronic pain and spasticity, with the first case performed in 1976 on a patient with arm pain following brachial plexus avulsion. In this surgery, the surgeon selectively destroys the posterolateral aspect of the spinal cord, corresponding to the area through which dorsal (sensory) root fibers enter the cord itself. The lesions are usually performed from one or two dermatomal levels above the level of the injury to one segment below it. Newer techniques including intramedullary monitoring have increased the success rate of DREZ therapy.

The benefit of this surgery is thought to be due to destruction of abnormal activity from neurons associated with pain in the dorsal horn, interruption of ascending afferent pathways, and rebalancing of the inhibitory and excitatory networks within a damaged sensory pathway. Surgical resection, radiofrequency, and laser have all been used to perform DREZ lesions. Currently, indications for DREZ lesions include brachial plexus avulsion, spinal cord/cauda equina lesions, pain due to syringomyelia, peripheral nerve lesions, postherpetic pain, and hyperspasticity.

Sympathectomy

Sympathectomy is a surgical procedure that is used to destroy nerves in the sympathetic system. By destroying these nerves, there is an increase in blood flow corresponding to the distribution of that nerve and a blockade of the sympathetically mediated pain response. Initially, a sympathetic block is done in order to determine whether the pain is amenable to blockade of these pathways, if so, the more definitive resection of the corresponding sympathetic ganglia is performed. This therapy is currently used for hyperhidrosis, complex regional pain syndrome (CRPS), and vasculitis. The surgery may be done either through an open technique or endoscopically guided. Complications can include neuralgias, Horner's syndrome, pneumothorax, ileus, and ejaculatory dysfunction. Efficacy can be up to 90% for the treatment of hyperhidrosis and up to 75% for the treatment of CRPS.

Midline Myelotomy

Early observations after lesioning of the central spinal cord showed analgesic effects for visceral pain, neuropathic pain in the upper and lower extremities, and central pain. The target area is typically the center of the spinal cord and anterior to the posterior funniculus. The pathophysiology is uncertain, however may involve the following explanations:

- Interruption of the polysynaptic pain pathways ascending into the gray matter
- Interruption of the spinothalamic tract
- Interruption of the juxtamidline fibers of the posterior column

Ideal patients include those with cancer in the abdominal or pelvic regions or with malignancy involving the lower trunk or lower extremities. Some have also postulated that this procedure may be useful for central pain states. Side effects include sensory impairment, paresis, and gait disturbances.

Percutaneous Cordotomy

This technique employs a lesion in the lateral spinothalamic tract in the anterolateral spinal cord. Patients that respond best to this procedure usually

- Over time, neurosurgical techniques have become more sophisticated, and there are now multiple modalities being used to treat similar pain states.
- Patient selection is critical when determining which neurosurgical technique to employ for treatment of pain. Neuropathic pain is best treated using these techniques.
- Spinal cord stimulator placement is now becoming more prolific. Those who tend to respond most favorably to SCS include those suffering from failed back syndrome, ischemic pain of peripheral vascular disease, angina pectoris, diabetic neuropathy, brachial plexus avulsion, cervical rhizopathy, CRPS I and II, postherpetic neuralgia, phantom limb syndrome, or cancer pain.

Further Reading

Dormont D, Seidenwurm D, et al. Neuroimaging and deep brain stimulation. *Am J Neuroradiol* 2010;31:15-23.

Giller Cole A. The neurosurgical treatment of pain. *Arch Neurol* 2003;60:1537-1540.

Lee A, Pititsis J. Spinal cord stimulation: indications and outcomes. *Neurosurg Focus* 2006;21:1-6.

Levy R, Deer T, Henderson J. Intracranial neurostimulation for pain control: A review. *Pain Physician* 2010;13:157-165.

Nicolaidis S. Neurosurgical treatments of intractable pain. *Metabolism* 2010; (59): S27-S31.

Wallace BA, Ashkan K, Benabid AL. Deep brain stimulation for the treatment of chronic, intractable pain. *Neurosurg Clin N Am* 2004;15:343-357.

A 48-year-old gentleman presents with a 25-year history of low back pain with radiation into his bilateral lower extremities. His pain began when he was delivering a refrigerator on a hand truck. The hand truck started to tip over and he strained his back trying to keep the hand truck upright. One year later he was diagnosed with a herniated disk and underwent an L4-5 laminectomy. He was reoperated on approximately one year later with persistent pain and at that time underwent a fusion. He has been disabled since the time of his injury for intractable low back and lower extremity pain.

He has been treated with every conceivable treatment including behavioral medicine, physical medicine, injection therapy, antidepressants, anticonvulsants, nonsteroidal anti-inflammatory drugs, opioids, and a trial with a spinal cord stimulating device. At the time of presentation, he was changing a 100 microgram fentanyl patch every 3 days and taking 16 milligrams of hydromorphone three times a day as needed. He states that he has begun using marijuana and finds that it is extremely useful in helping to control his pain. He lives in a state with medical marijuana legislation and specifically requests that I prescribe or recommend the use of marijuana for his pain.

What do you do now?

This patient's history is not unusual. He suffers from intractable chronic pain refractory to all known therapies. His opioid doses are extremely high. The ratio of morphine equivalents to hydromorphone is 7.5 to 1 such that his 16 milligrams of hydromorphone is equivalent to 120 milligrams of morphine three times a day. His 100 microgram fentanyl patch is roughly equivalent to 300 milligrams per day of oral morphine. His daily opioid dosage is then equivalent to approximately 660 morphine equivalents per day, far higher than what is considered the "inside the box dosage" of 200 milligrams per day of morphine equivalents.

This patient has recently relocated to the State of Vermont, where there is medical marijuana legislation. There is currently medical marijuana legislation in 12 states within the United States; these include Washington, Oregon, California, Nevada, Montana, Colorado, New Mexico, Alaska, Hawaii, Maine, Vermont, and Maryland.

Six other states are considering medical marijuana, and medical marijuana has been rejected in only one state and, that is South Dakota. There are reports that there may be 20,000 authorized medical cannabis users in the State of Washington alone. A recent survey in Canada has shown that 10% of patients with chronic, noncancer pain currently use marijuana for pain relief.

This patient asks specifically that his doctor recommends or prescribes marijuana to him. The consideration here is that the physician's Drug Enforcement Agency (DEA) license is provided by the federal government and the federal government still considers marijuana an unscheduled drug, meaning that there is no medical indication. The federal government thus has the ability to remove the physician's DEA license if he or she recommends the use of marijuana. The Vermont Medical Society, for example, considered this to be an extremely important issue in helping to draft the legislation in that state permitting the usage of medical marijuana. Legislation varies from state to state, and in the State of Vermont a patient who wishes to obtain a medical marijuana "card" can go online and obtain an application from the Commissioner of Health for the State of Vermont. The patient can then complete a form, a portion of which is completed by his physician. The physician does not recommend or prescribe marijuana, but simply attests to the fact that the patient has a bona fide physician-patient relationship, which must have lasted at least a minimum of six months and requires that a complete history and physical examination have been performed. The physician will then attest to the fact that the patient suffers from a specific condition making him or her eligible to receive a medical marijuana "card" from the State of Vermont.

There is an expanding body of evidence supporting the efficacy of marijuana in treating a variety of pain conditions. Unfortunately, provider, patient, and societal bias with regard to this issue is rampant and while studies of efficacy have begun to be published, there is little safety data with regard to inhaled marijuana, which in the United States must be obtained from an unregulated source.

Proponents of medical cannabis site its safety, but there are clearly uncertainties regarding safety, composition, and dosage. In France, the Department of Health has advised cannabis smokers of the respiratory risks associated with the common practice of sellers of marijuana adding glass beads or sand to cannabis in order to increase its weight. Cannabis has been linked to elevated rates of myocardial infarction and cardiac arrhythmias and it has been implicated in the occurrence of depression, anxiety, psychosis, bipolar disorder, and amotivational state. It has teratogenic affects on the developing perinatal brain. It is associated with chronic bronchitis, reduced lung density, and has been linked to cancers at eight sites. The evidence supporting all of these risks is controversial. The real risk may or may not be ultimately proven or disproven. Patients can minimize the carcinogenic and respiratory risks by using vaporizers. There is clearly, at this time, evidence of abuse, misuse, and addiction. Evidence-based guidelines do not exist to guide practitioners in the usage of medical cannabis, but physicians are commonly asked to at least tacitly condone the use of medical marijuana.

HOW SHOULD THE PHYSICIAN MANAGE THIS PATIENT?

If the physician has a bona fide relationship with the patient and can attest to that the patient suffers a painful condition, the physician may make this attestation without jeopardizing his or her license. It is important for the physician to clearly describe the potential risks of using inhaled marijuana or cannabis as I have described above and to document this discussion. There is insufficient efficacy or safety data to support the use of marijuana in the developing brain. Patients need to be motivated to attend school or work, and marijuana may make this impossible. Patients who are responsible for other individuals, or who engage in dangerous occupations, or use dangerous equipment such as chainsaws or circular saws may not be able to use marijuana safely.

The attestation of a patient's medical condition permitting him or her to obtain medical marijuana or cannabis should not be a responsibility undertaken lightly by the physician, since there are potentially severe risks associated with the use of this drug that our patients should be warned about. Treatment should be based on a trial with specific goals predefined such as, in the case of this patient, a reduction of opioid dose to below 200 mg of morphine equivalents per day. Reduction in pain scores and improvement in functionality should also be a requirement for continued attestation to the presence of a condition permitting the use of this drug. If the use of marijuana is "medicalized," then the rules surrounding a potentially dangerous and addictive drug should be followed.

KEY POINTS TO REMEMBER

- Marijuana or medical cannabis may be a useful drug to treat pain, but side effects and adverse effects are poorly described at this time.
- Providers should be careful not to jeopardize their DEA privileges by "recommending" or "prescribing" medical cannabis.
- The potential risks and benefits should be discussed with the patient in detail and documented in the medical record.
- Treatment should be a trial with continued use contingent on prespecified goals of therapy.

Further Reading

Aggarwal SK, Carter GT, Sullivan MD, et al. Characteristics of patients with chronic pain accessing treatment with medical cannabis in Washington State. *J Opioid Manag* 2009;5(5):257-286.

Cohen PJ. Medical marijuana: the conflict between scientific evidence and political ideology. *J Pain Palliat Care Pharmacother* 2009;23(1):4-25.

Delourme J, Delattre C, Godard P, et al. Respiratory consequences of inhalation of adulterated cannabis [in French]. *Rev Mal Respir* 2009;26(5):552-556.

Fanciullo GJ. Medical cannabis. *J Opioid Manag* 2009;5(5):245-246.

Filbey FM, Schacht JP, Myers US, et al. Marijuana craving in the brain. *Proc Natl Acad Sci U S A* 2009;106(31):13016-13021.

Lynch ME, Young J, Clark AJ. Clinical note: a case series of patients using medicinal marihuana for management of chronic pain under the Canadian marihuana medical access regulations. *J Pain Sympt Manage* 2006;32(5):497-501.

McCarberg BH, Barkin RL. The future of cannibinoids as analgesic agents: a pharmacologic, pharmacokinetic, and pharmacodynamics overview. *Am J Ther* 2007;14(5):475-483.

Reece AS. Chronic toxicology of cannabis. *Clin Toxicol* 2009;47(6):517-524.

Ware MA, Doyle CR, Woods R, et al. Cannabis use for chronic non-cancer pain: results of a prospective study. *Pain* 2003;102:211-216.

Wilsey B, Marcotte T, Tsodikov A, et al. A randomized, placebo-controlled, crossover trial of cannabis cigarettes in neuropathic pain. *J Pain* 2008;9(6):506-521.

Index

ablative neurosurgical procedures
  dorsal root entry zone lesions, 158
  dorsal root ganglionectomy, 158
  midline myelotomy, 159
  percutaneous cordotomy, 159–160
  peripheral neurectomy, 157, 158
  sympathectomy, 159
acetaminophen
  for radiculopathy, 37
  for spinal cord injury, pain, 66
acetazolamide, for MS-related pain, 31, 33
acupuncture
  for arachnoiditis, 86
  for brachial plexus injury, 44
  for phantom pain, 64
  for supraorbital neuralgia, 76
acute pain syndromes (table), 31
acyclovir, for Ramsay Hunt syndrome, 72
addictive disorder and chronic pain, 109–112
  case presentation, 109
  drug usage/abuse survey, 110–111
  opioid use/abuse data, 111
  risk stratification for patients, 110
alpha-2 adrenergic agonists (A2A), 144–145
amantadine, for MS-related pain, 31, 33
American Society of Addiction Medicine,
    110
amitriptyline
  for central post-stroke pain, 24–25
  for diabetic peripheral neuropathy, 14
  for MS-related pain, 32
  for postherpetic neuralgia, 19
  side effects of, 139
  starting dose/dosage range, 129
  for tension headaches, 127
amputation of limbs. See phantom pain
analgesics, intrathecal, 67. See also
    bupivacaine; clonidine;
    hydromorphone; morphine

anesthetics. See also bupivacaine; lidocaine;
    mexiletine
  for central post-stroke pain, 25–26
  for MS-related pain, 31, 32–33
anticonvulsants, 131–136. See also
    carbamazepine; gabapentin;
    lamotrigine; oxcarbazepine;
    phenytoin; pregabalin; topiramate;
    valproic acid; zonisamide
  for arachnoiditis, 86
  for brachial plexus injuries, 44
  case presentation, 131
  for central post-stroke pain, 25
  for complex regional pain syndrome, 7
  for dental pain, 55
  for diabetic peripheral neuropathy, 14
  for glossopharyngeal neuralgia, 81
  mechanisms of action, 132
    not voltage-gated sodium channels,
      134t, 135–136
    voltage-gated sodium channel, 132,
      133, 134t, 135
  for mononeuropathies, 101
  for MS-related pain, 31
  NNT analgesia confidence interval, 133
  for postherpetic neuralgia, 19
  for spinal cord injury, pain, 67
  starting doses/dosages, 134
  for supraorbital neuralgia, 76
antidepressants, 125–130. See also
    citalopram; fluvoxamine; selective
    serotonin reuptake inhibitors;
    tricyclic antidepressants
  adjuvant analgesic role, 126
  approach to therapy with, 128, 130
  case presentation, 125
  for central post-stroke pain, 24–25
  for complex regional pain syndrome, 7
  for dental pain, 55

for depression with chronic pain, 107
for diabetic peripheral neuropathy, 14
for glossopharyngeal neuralgia, 81
for mononeuropathies, 101
for spinal cord injury, pain, 67
starting doses/dosage range, 129
arachnoiditis, 83–87
case presentation, 83
description, 84
diagnostic criteria, 85
management
nonpharmacologic, 86
pharmacologic, 86
procedural/surgical, 86–87
signs and symptoms, 84–85
atypical face pain, 60–61
baclofen
intrathecal, for spinal cord injury, 67
for MS-related pain, 31, 33
for spinal cord injury, pain, 67
for trigeminal neuralgia, 59
beta blockers, for phantom pain, 64
biofeedback
for arachnoiditis, 86
for brachial plexus injury, 44
botulinum toxin injections
for occipital neuralgia, 91
for spinal cord injury, pain, 67
brachial plexus injury, 39–44
anatomy (brachial plexus), 42
case presentation, 39
diagnostic criteria, 40, 41
epidemiology of, 40
investigative testing
electrophysiology, 43
histamine test, 43
radiographic images, 42, 43
Leffert classification, 41
management
nonpharmacologic, 44
pharmacologic, 43–44
procedural/surgical, 44
bupivacaine

for MS-related pain, 31
for spinal cord injury, pain, 67
buprenorphine, for addictive disorder with
chronic pain, 111
calcitonin, for phantom pain, 64
cancer pain, 94–96
in breast cancer survivors, 95–96
case presentation, 94
interdisciplinary paradigms, 96
posttreatment, postsurgical pain
syndromes, 95
psychological coping strategies, 96
radiation-induced plexopathy, 96
capsaicin, topical, 64, 146
carbamazepine
for central post-stroke pain, 25
for glossopharyngeal neuralgia, 81
mechanism of action, side-effects, 132
for MS-related pain, 31
NNT analgesia confidence interval, 133
for postherpetic neuralgia, 19
starting dose/dosage range, 134t
for trigeminal neuralgia, 31, 59
carbonic anhydrase inhibitors, 33. See also
acetazolamide
case presentation
arachnoiditis, 83
brachial plexus injury, 39
central post-stroke pain, 22
complex regional pain syndrome, 3
depression and chronic pain, 105
glossopharyngeal neuralgia, 79
mononeuropathy, 98
multiple sclerosis-related pain, 29
and neurosurgical procedures for pain,
155
occipital neuralgia, 89
opioid use, 138
peripheral neuropathy, 10
phantom pain, 62
post-thoracotomy pain, 49
postherpetic neuralgia, 16
radiculopathy, 35

Ramsay Hunt syndrome, 69
spinal cord injury and pain, 65
superficial radial nerve injury, 46
trigeminal neuralgia, 57
causalgia (CRPS Type II), 4
central post-stroke pain (CPSP), 22–27
case presentation, 22
diagnostic criteria, 24
management
nonpharmacologic, 26
pharmacologic, 24–26, 133
procedural/surgical, 26–27
secondary causes, 24
signs and symptoms, 23
chronic pain syndromes (table), 31
citalopram, for central post-stroke pain, 25
clonidine
mechanism of action, side-effects,
144–145
for spinal cord injury, pain, 67
codeine phosphate, for CPSP, 26
cognitive behavioral therapy (CBT)
for arachnoiditis, 86
for depression with chronic pain, 107,
126
for hypochondriasis, 116
for supraorbital neuralgia, 76
complex regional pain syndrome (CRPS),
3–8
alternate names, 4
case presentation, 3
diagnostic criteria
stages 1–3 (description), 6
subtypes, 7
management
nonpharmacologic, 7
pharmacologic, 7–8
procedural/surgical treatment, 8
overdiagnosis potential, 4
vasomotor/sudomotor dysfunction,
edema, 5f
conversion disorder, 117
CPSP. See central post-stroke pain

CRPS Type I (reflex sympathetic
dystrophy), 4
CRPS Type II (causalgia), 4
CT (computed tomography)
for arachnoiditis, 85
for CPSP, 24
for occipital neuralgia, 91
for post-thoracotomy pain, 51
deep brain stimulation (DBS)
for central post-stroke pain, 26
for spinal cord injury, pain, 67
dental pain, 53–55
case presentation, 53
management
mental health treatment, 55
peripheral nerve stimulation, 55
pharmacologic, 55
physical therapy, 55
signs and symptoms, 54
depression and chronic pain, 105–108
case presentation, 105
influence on disabilities, 106
management
nonpharmacologic, 107
pharmacologic, 107
procedural/surgical, 108
underdiagnosis/undertreatment of, 107
desipramine
amitriptyline comparison, 19
for diabetic peripheral neuropathy, 14
starting dose/dosage range, 129
dextromethorphan
for central post-stroke pain, 26
mechanism of action, 145–146
diabetes, 0000
diabetic amyotrophy, 99
diabetic mononeuropathy, 99
diabetic peripheral neuropathy (DPN), 13
diagnostic criteria
for arachnoiditis, 85
for brachial plexus injury, 40, 41
for central post-stroke pain, 24
for complex regional pain syndrome, 4–7

for occipital neuralgia, 91
for pain disorder, 115–116
for peripheral neuropathy, 11
post-thoracotomy pain, 51
for postherpetic neuralgia, 17
for Ramsay Hunt syndrome, 71–72
for trigeminal neuralgia, 58
difficult chronic pain patients, 119–122
case presentation, 119–120
"hateful patient"/"entitled demander"
types, 121
noncompliance/dissatisfaction of, 121
physician strategies, 121–122
dorsal root entry zone (DREZ) lesions, 158
dorsal root ganglionectomy, 158
Drug Abuse Warning Network, 111
duloxetine
for complex regional pain syndrome, 7
for dental pain, 55
for diabetic peripheral neuropathy, 14
for neuropathic pain syndrome, 47, 128
starting dose/dosage range, 129
dysesthetic pain (in MS), 30
baclofen (oral/intrathecal) treatment, 33
lamotrigine treatment, 32
octreotide treatment, 33
electromyography (EMG)
for brachial plexus injuries, 43
for peripheral neuropathy diagnosis, 11
for Ramsay Hunt syndrome, 71
"entitled demander" (difficult patient type),
121
entrapment syndromes, 0000, 100
epidemiology
of brachial plexus injury, 40
of glossopharyngeal neuralgia, 80
of postherpetic neuralgia, 17
of radiculopathy, 36
of trigeminal neuralgia, 58
exposure therapy, for PTSD, 115
fluoxetine
side effects of, 128
starting dose/dosage range, 129

fluvoxamine (SSRI), for CPSP, 25, 27
gabapentin
for central post-stroke pain, 25, 27
for complex regional pain syndrome, 7,
136
for dental pain, 55
for diabetic peripheral neuropathy, 14
interactions, 136
mechanism of action, side-effects,
135–136
for MS-related pain, 31, 32
for neuropathic pain syndrome, 47
NNT analgesia confidence interval, 133
for phantom pain, 63
for postherpetic neuralgia, 19, 136
for supraorbital neuralgia, 76
for trigeminal neuralgia, 59
geniculate neuralgia. See Ramsay Hunt
syndrome
glossopharyngeal neuralgia (GN), 79–81
case presentation, 79
diagnostic criteria, 80
epidemiology, 80
management
pharmacologic, 31, 80–81
surgical, 81
prognosis, 81
signs and symptoms, 80
"hateful patient" (difficult patient type),
121
histamine test, for brachial plexus injuries,
43
HIV (human immunodeficiency virus), 133
Horner's syndrome, 41
hydrocodone, use/abuse data, 111
hydromorphone
morphine equivalents, 164
for spinal cord injury, pain, 67
hypnosis
for arachnoiditis, 86
for brachial plexus injury, 44
for phantom pain, 64
hypochondriasis, 116

inflammatory lesions (of MS), 30
International Association for the Study of
    Pain (IASP)
    CRPS diagnostic criteria, 4
    "pain" definition, 50, 106
    trigeminal neuralgia definition, 58
International Headache Society (IHS), 90
ketamine
    for central post-stroke pain, 26
    for CRPS, 8
    mechanism of action, 145
    for phantom pain, 64
lamotrigine
    for central post-stroke pain, 25
    for diabetic peripheral neuropathy, 14
    mechanism of action, side-effects, 133
    for MS-related pain, 31, 32
    starting dose/dosage range, 134
    for trigeminal neuralgia, 59, 133
Leffert classification, of brachial plexus
    injuries, 41
levorphanol (oral), for CPSP, 26
L'hermitte's sign (in MS), 30
    carbamazepine treatment, 31
    lidocaine treatment, 32
    mexiletine treatment, 32
lidocaine
    for central post-stroke pain, 25–26, 27
    for diabetic peripheral neuropathy, 14
    for MS-related pain, 31, 32
    for postherpetic neuralgia, 18
Lidoderm Patch' for postherpetic neuralgia,
    18
limb amputation. See phantom pain
local anesthetics (LAs). See also bupivacaine;
    lidocaine; mexiletine
    for glossopharyngeal neuralgia, 80
    mechanism of action, 144
    for MS-related pain, 31, 32
    for occipital neuralgia, 91, 92
    for post-thoracotomy pain, 51
    for postherpetic neuralgia, 18
    for superficial radial nerve injury, 47

for supraorbital neuralgia, 76
lumbar arachnoiditis. See arachnoiditis
lumbar nerve syndromes, 37t
massage
    for arachnoiditis pain, 86
    for phantom pain, 64
medical cannabis
    case presentation, 163
    licensing issues, 164–165
    physician management guidelines,
        165–166
    safety, composition, dosage concerns,
        165
    states with/considering legislation, 164
    use data, 110
methadone
    analgesic duration/half-life, 139–140
    for CRPS, 7
    for diabetic peripheral neuropathy, 14
    use/abuse data, 111
methylprednisolone
    for MS-related pain, 32
    for Ramsey Hunt syndrome, 72
mexiletine
    for central post-stroke pain, 27
    for MS-related pain, 31, 32
    treatment efficacies, 144
milnacipran, for central post-stroke pain, 26
misoprostol, for MS-related pain, 31, 33
mononeuritis multiplex, 99–100
mononeuropathy, 98–101
    case presentation, 98
    management, 101
    types of
        diabetic, 99
        entrapment neuropathies, 100
        mononeuritis multiplex, 99–100
        peripheral nerve tumors, 101
morphine
    for central post-stroke pain, 26
    for diabetic peripheral neuropathy, 14
    hydromorphone equivalents, 164
    for spinal cord injury, pain, 67

Morton's neuralgia, 100
motor cortex stimulation (MCS) procedure, 26, 161
MRI (magnetic resonance imaging)
  for arachnoiditis, 85
  for atypical face pain, 60–61
  for central post-stroke pain, 24
  for entrapment neuropathies, 100
  for low-back/radicular pain, 38
  for occipital neuralgia, 91
  for post-thoracotomy pain, 51
multiple sclerosis-related pain, 29–33
  case presentation, 29
  inflammatory lesions, 30
  management
    pharmacologic, 31–33
    procedural/surgical treatment, 33
muscle relaxants. *See also* tizanidine
  for glossopharyngeal neuralgia, 81
  for spinal cord injury, 66
naloxone, for central post-stroke pain, 26
nerve conduction studies (NCS)
  for brachial plexus injuries, 43
  for cancer patients, 96
  for peripheral neuropathy, 11
  for Ramsay Hunt syndrome, 71
neuropathic pain (in MS), 30
neurosurgical procedures for pain, 155–161
  ablative techniques
    dorsal root entry zone lesions, 158
    dorsal root ganglionectomy, 158
    midline myelotomy, 159
    percutaneous cordotomy, 159–160
    peripheral neurectomy, 157, 158
    sympathectomy, 159
  case presentation, 155
  classification of techniques, 157t
  indications
    neuropathic pain, 156
    nociceptive pain, 156–157
  non-ablative procedures
    deep brain stimulation, 26, 67, 160–161

motor cortex stimulation, 161
NMDA receptor antagonists. *See also* ketamine
  for central post-stroke syndrome, 26
  mechanism of action, 145–146
  for phantom pain, 64
non-ablative neurosurgical procedures
  deep brain stimulation, 26, 67, 160–161
  motor cortex stimulation, 161
nonpharmacologic management
  of arachnoiditis, 86
  of brachial plexus injuries, 44
  of central post-stroke pain, 26
  of complex regional pain syndrome, 7
  of depression, chronic pain, 107
  of phantom pain, 64
  of postherpetic neuralgia, 18
  of spinal cord injury, 67
  of supraorbital neuralgia, 76
nonsteroidal anti-inflammatory drugs (NSAIDs) treatment
  for arachnoiditis, 86
  for brachial plexus injury, 44
  for complex regional pain syndrome, 7
  for depression with chronic pain, 108
  for neuropathic pain syndrome, 47
  for spinal cord injury, pain, 66
nortriptyline
  amitriptyline comparison, 19
  for diabetic peripheral neuropathy, 14
  starting dose/dosage range, 129
occipital neuralgia, 89–92
  case presentation, 89
  causes of, 90
  description, 90
  diagnostic criteria, 91
  treatment, 91–92
octreotide, for MS-related pain, 31, 33
opioids, 138–142. *See also* levorphanol; methadone; morphine; naloxone; tramadol
  for arachnoiditis, 86
  for brachial plexus injuries, 44

case presentation, 138
for central post-stroke pain, 26
for dental pain, 55
for depression with chronic pain, 108
for diabetic peripheral neuropathy, 14
intrathecal, for phantom pain, 64
misuse, by difficult patients, 121
for neuropathic pain syndrome, 47
for postherpetic neuralgia, 19
prescription monitoring, 141–142
for radiculopathy, 37
side effects of, 140–141
for spinal cord injury, pain, 67
use/abuse data, 111
optic neuritis, steroid therapy for, 32
oxcarbazepine
mechanism of action, 133
starting dose/dosage range, 134
for trigeminal neuralgia, 59
oxycodone
for diabetic peripheral neuropathy, 14
for radiculopathy, 37
use/abuse data, 111
OxyContin, use/abuse data, 110
pain disorder, 115–116
Parkinson's disease, 33, 156
paroxetine
for PTSD, 115
starting dose/dosage range, 129
paroxysmal limb pain
carbamazepine treatment, 31
lamotrigine treatment, 32
lidocaine treatment, 32
mexiletine treatment, 32
phenytoin treatment, 32
TCA treatment, 32
patients that are difficult. See difficult
chronic pain patients
percutaneous cordotomy, 159–160
peripheral nerve stimulation (PNS),
151–153
indications, 55, 151
outcomes, 152

trial and implantation, 152
peripheral neurectomy, 157, 158
peripheral neuropathy, 10–15
case presentation, 10
diagnostic criteria, 11
differential diagnosis, symmetric
polyneuropathies, 12t
initial assessment of pain, 13
management, 12, 13
pharmacologic treatment, 14, 14t, 132
procedural/surgical treatment, 14, 15
symptoms/definitions, 13t
persistent post-thoracotomy pain syndrome
(PTPS), 50. See also post-
thoracotomy pain (acute/chronic)
personality disorders, 117
phantom pain, 62–64
case presentation, 62
description/mechanism, 63
management
nonpharmacologic, 64
pharmacologic, 63–64
pharmacologic management
of addictive disorder, chronic pain, 111
of arachnoiditis, 86
of brachial plexus injury, 43–44
of central post-stroke pain, 24–26
of complex regional pain syndrome, 7–8
of dental pain, 55
of depression, chronic pain, 107
of multiple sclerosis-related pain, 31–33
of peripheral neuropathy, 14, 14t
of phantom pain, 63–64
of post-thoracotomy pain, 51–52
of postherpetic neuralgia, 18–20
of spinal cord injury and pain, 66–67
of superficial radial nerve injury, 47
of supraorbital neuralgia, 76
of trigeminal neuralgia, 31, 33, 59–60
phenytoin
for central post-stroke pain, 25
for MS-related pain, 31, 32
NNT analgesia confidence interval, 133

for trigeminal neuralgia, 59
physical therapy
  for arachnoiditis, 86
  for complex regional pain syndrome, 7, 8
  for dental pain, 55
  for MS-related pain, 30
  for phantom pain, 64
  for radiculopathy, 36, 37
post-thoracotomy pain (acute/chronic),
    49–52
  case presentation, 49
  diagnostic criteria, 51
  IASP definition, 50
  intraoperative factors leading to, 50
  pharmacologic treatment, 51–52
  targeted treatment periods, 50
post-traumatic stress disorder (PTSD),
    114–115
postherpetic neuralgia, 16–20
  case presentation, 16
  diagnostic criteria, 17
  epidemiology of, 17
  management
    nonpharmacologic, 18
    pharmacologic, 18–20
  signs and symptoms, 17–18
postherpetic neuralgia (PHN), 17
prednisone, side effects of, 139
pregabalin
  for dental pain, 55
  for diabetic peripheral neuropathy, 14,
    136
  mechanism of action, side-effects, 136
  for neuropathic pain syndrome, 47
  for postherpetic neuralgia, 136
  for supraorbital neuralgia, 76
procedural treatment
  for arachnoiditis, 86–87
  for brachial plexus injuries, 44
  for central post-stroke pain, 26–27
  for complex regional pain syndrome, 8
  of depression, chronic pain, 108
  for multiple sclerosis-related pain, 33

for peripheral neuropathy, 14, 15
for postherpetic neuralgia, 18
for supraorbital neuralgia, 76
for trigeminal neuralgia, 60
propofol, for central post-stroke pain, 27
psychiatric disorders and chronic pain,
    113–117
  case presentation, 113
  post-traumatic stress disorder, 114–115
  somatoform disorders
    conversion disorder, 117
    hypochondriasis, 116
    pain disorder, 115–116
    personality disorders, 117
    somatoform disorder, 116–117
psychological treatment. See also cognitive
    behavioral therapy
  for cancer pain, 96
  for depression with chronic pain, 107
radiation-induced plexopathy, 96
radiculopathy, 35–38
  case presentation, 35
  epidemiology of, 36
  management of, 36, 37–38
  signs and symptoms, 36
Ramsay Hunt syndrome (geniculate
    neuralgia), 69–72
  case presentation, 69
  diagnostic criteria, 71–72
  management of, 72
  prognosis, 72
  signs and symptoms, 70–71
  types of, 70
reflex sympathetic dystrophy (RSD), 4
repetitive transcranial magnetic stimulation
    (rTMS), for CPSP, 26
Rochester Diabetic Nephropathy Study, 11
selective norepinephrine reuptake inhibitors
    (SNRIs). See also duloxetine;
    venlafaxine
  for central post-stroke pain, 25
  for depression with chronic pain, 107
  for diabetic peripheral neuropathy, 14

mechanisms of action, uses, side effects, 128
selective serotonin reuptake inhibitors (SSRIs)
    advantages/benefits of, 127
    adverse side effects of, 127–128
    for central post-stroke pain, 25
    for depression with chronic pain, 107
    interactions with other medications, 128
    mechanisms of action, 128
sertraline
    for PTSD, 115
    starting dose/dosage range, 129
shingles (herpes zoster), 17
signs and symptoms
    arachnoiditis, 84–85
    central post-stroke pain, 23
    dental pain, 54
    glossopharyngeal neuralgia, 80
    postherpetic neuralgia, 17–18
    radiculopathy, 36
    Ramsay Hunt syndrome, 70–71
    supraorbital neuralgia, 75
sodium channel blockers, for phantom pain, 63
somatoform disorders
    conversion disorder, 117
    difficult patients with, 121
    hypochondriasis, 116
    pain disorder, 115–116
    personality disorders, 117
    somatoform disorder, 116–117
spinal cord injury and pain, 65–68
    case presentation, 65
    description, 66
    management
        nonpharmacologic, 67
        pharmacologic, 66–67
spinal cord stimulation (SCS)
    implantation decision criteria, 149
    indications, 18, 52, 67, 149
    neurostimulation principles, 151
    trial and implantation, 150–151

steroids
    for MS-related pain, 31, 32
    for neuropathic pain syndrome, 47
    for optic neuritis, 32
Substance Abuse and Mental Health Services Administration survey, 110–111
superficial radial nerve injury, 46–47
    case presentation, 46
    pharmacologic treatment, 47
supraorbital neuralgia, 74–76
    diagnostic criteria, 75
    management
        nonpharmacologic, 76
        pharmacologic, 76
        procedural/surgical, 76
    signs and symptoms, 75
surgical treatment. See also neurosurgical procedures for pain
    for arachnoiditis, 86–87
    for brachial plexus injury, 44
    for central post-stroke pain, 26–27
    for complex regional pain syndrome, 8
    of depression, chronic pain, 108
    for glossopharyngeal neuralgia, 81
    for multiple sclerosis-related pain, 33
    for peripheral neuropathy, 14, 15
    for phantom pain, 64
    for radiculopathy, 37–38
    for supraorbital neuralgia, 76
    for trigeminal neuralgia, 60
sympathectomy, 159
three-phase bone scintigraphy, for CRPS diagnosis, 6
tizanidine, 144–145
topical agents
    for diabetic peripheral neuropathy, 14
    for phantom limb pain, 64
    for postherpetic neuralgia, 18
    for PTPS, 51
    for superficial radial nerve injury, 47
    types of/mechanism of action, 146
topiramate

for central post-stroke pain, 25
for diabetic peripheral neuropathy, 14,
    135
interactions, 135
mechanism of action, 135
starting dose/dosage range, 134
for supraorbital neuralgia, 76
for trigeminal neuralgia, 59
tramadol
for central post-stroke pain, 26
for diabetic peripheral neuropathy, 14
transcutaneous electrical nerve stimulation
    (TENS)
for arachnoiditis, 86
for brachial plexus injury, 44
for phantom pain, 64
tricyclic antidepressants (TCAs). See also
    amitriptyline
adjuvant role of, 127
adverse side effects of, 127
for arachnoiditis, 86
for brachial plexus injury, 44
for central post-stroke pain, SSRIs
contraindications to use, 19
for depression with chronic pain, 107
for diabetic peripheral neuropathy, 14
elderly patients usage risks, 127
for MS-related pain, 31, 32
for occipital neuralgia, 91
for phantom pain, 63

for postherpetic neuralgia, 19
side effect profile, 60
for supraorbital neuralgia, 76
for trigeminal neuralgia, 59
trigeminal neuralgia (TN), 30, 57–60. See
    also atypical face pain
case presentation, 57
diagnostic criteria, 58
epidemiology of, 58
management
    pharmacologic, 31, 33, 59–60, 132
    procedural/surgical, 60
secondary causes of, 59
ultrasound, for phantom pain, 64
valproate, diabetic peripheral neuropathy,
    14
valproic acid
mechanism of action, side-effects, 135
starting dose/dosage range, 134t
varicella zoster virus, 17, 17
venlafaxine
for diabetic peripheral neuropathy, 14
starting dose/dosage range, 129
vestibulocochlear stimulation, for CPSP, 26
video-assisted thoracic surgery (VATS),
    50–51
Zanaflex, for spinal cord injury, 67
zonisamide
for central post-stroke pain, 25
for trigeminal neuralgia, 59